The QUANTUM *Psychiatrist*

The QUANTUM *Psychiatrist*

From Zero to Zen Using Evidence-Based Solutions Beyond Medication and Therapy

Dr. Dona Biswas

No problem can be solved from the
same level of consciousness that created it.

—Albert Einstein

For more information, address: quantumpsychiatrist@gmail.com

FIRST EDITION

ISBN-13: 978-0-6488651-0-0

www.thequantumpsychiatrist.com

DOWNLOAD THE QUANTUM MEDITATIONS FREE!

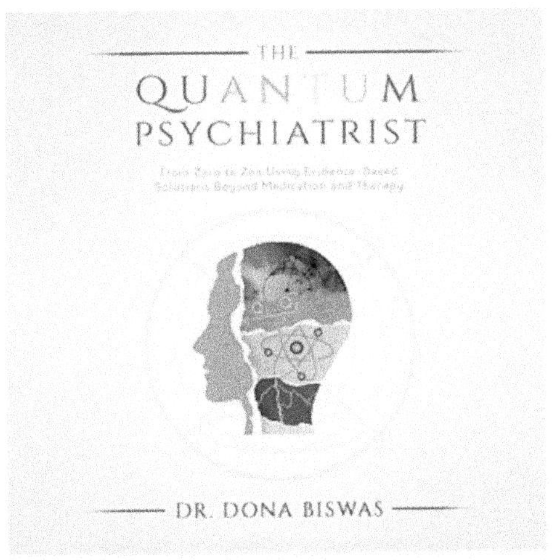

READ THIS FIRST

Just to say thank you for buying my book,
I would like to give you the mp3 version of
my Quantum Meditations 100% FREE!

TO DOWNLOAD GO TO:

https://thequantumpsychiatrist.com/free-gift/

For my parents, who taught me how to dream.

ACKNOWLEDGEMENTS

There are so many people that I want to acknowledge that I fear even a book is not enough to cover them all, but I will do my best. First of all, I would like to acknowledge all the original thinkers of integrative medicine who have paved the path for the future. They include Dr. Deepak Chopra, Dr. Bernie Siegal, Dr. Larry Dossey, Dr Wayne Dyer, Dr. Andrew Weil, among many others.

I would like to thank those psychiatrists whose thoughts have helped me think outside the box: Dr. Norman Doidge, Dr. Bessel van der Kolk, Dr. Judith Orloff and others. Your work inspired me to seek solutions beyond medications and psychotherapy.

I would also like to thank those practitioners of energy psychology whose work I have referred to in my book: Dr. Church Dawson, Dr. Joe Dispenza, Gregg Braden, Dr James Oschmann, and others.

A special word of thanks to Professor Amit Goswami, whose books and course on "Quantum Psychology" helped me integrate my understanding of quantum physics and whose model I have relied on to explore different modalities of healing.

A big thank you to my clients, whose journeys have inspired me to write this book and I hope it makes a difference in their lives, as their lives have made a difference to mine.

My heartfelt thanks and dedication goes to my father, who forged a new career at the age of 58 and still inspires my 'can do' attitude, and my mother, who is my emotional rock. And finally, a big thanks to my daughter and my husband, who patiently endured my mood swings and long absences during the writing of this book.

—Dr. Dona Biswas

CONTENTS

PART 3: BACK TO THE FUTURE

Introduction

THE JOURNEY BEGINS

"The only thing that interferes with my learning is my education."

—Albert Einstein

A fundamental paradigm shift is sweeping the world of medicine today: Quantum Psychiatry is one such paradigm. This new paradigm is based on the principles of quantum physics, which acknowledges the primacy of consciousness. In other words, the brain does not produce consciousness, as consciousness is everywhere. Quantum psychiatry recognizes that we are multidimensional beings and thus healing should be multidimensional as well.

I have been interested in holistic approaches to health since my teenage years, as a result of personal experience. Toward the end of high school, I developed a severe, debilitating asthma and was in bed for the better part of the school year. My father, frustrated by fruitless trips to the doctor and sleepless nights, took me to a homeopath, who prescribed a combination of medicines which ultimately reduced my asthmatic attacks drastically. As a result, I was able to pursue with the grind of medical school. However, not once during all my academic journeys did I hear any mention of alternative healing modalities without the ideas being immediately labelled as quackery.

Thanks to my personal healing experience through homeopathy, I was convinced that we were barking up the wrong tree and abandoning something worthy of more research.

During my internship, I burnt the midnight oil, reading as much as I could in between clinical duties and studying to get into a postgraduate course. I was torn between two disciplines which intrigued me: psychiatry and general medicine. Psychiatry I considered to be the frontier of medicine, containing the most likely possibility of progress and research in the coming decades.

I soon discovered the works of Herbert Benson, Deepak Chopra, Andrew Weil, Larry Dossey, and Bernie Siegel, amongst many other crusaders of Mind-Body Medicine. Mind-body medicine was an emerging discipline which blended a mish-mash of complementary medicine, lifestyle interventions, and psychoneuroimmunology (how the mind influences hormones and immunity). These pioneers, through various examples of spontaneous healing, described the role of *intention* in healing.

Finally, I had found other people who saw the importance in alternative medicine, like I did.

However, I was left with unanswered questions and a sense of incompleteness, like I was still only seeing some parts of the picture.

For instance, the placebo response was intriguing to say the least. The placebo response occurs when a person who is sick begins to heal after they believe they are given a treatment, even if that treatment was nothing but sugar pills. The placebo response is so ubiquitous in nature that all rigorous drug trials are required to have a placebo arm in order to demonstrate clear superiority of the trial medication to a placebo. In depression research, placebo responses are as high as 30% while conventional antidepressant medications demonstrate response rates around 60%. One third of people with depression are able to get better with a placebo alone! That alone speaks volume for the potential for self-healing in medicine.

What then is the mechanism of the placebo response? How does it work? I wondered if it were possible to harness the power of the placebo response consciously, and what that could do for medicine as a whole. Most researchers have ignored this question, considering the placebo response as only an inconvenient factor in research. But what if we had a clear mechanism worked out? Perhaps more and more people would be able to heal themselves! What an exciting possibility!

An interesting episode I still remember from my year of internship at a public hospital, is a reflection of the mechanistic viewpoint that medicine is deeply entrenched in. I was sitting in the doctors' room during my lunch break, reading Deepak Chopra's *Quantum Healing,* a fascinating account of the role of consciousness in healing. One of the "real" doctors came into the room, eyed my book and, curling the corner of his lips, said, "Don't tell me you believe in that crap!"

Confronted by such a statement, I mumbled something and quickly stuffed my book into my bag, away from prying eyes, deciding in that instant to keep my private research to myself till I had something more substantial to say.

Unable to find convincing answers in my scientific textbooks, I turned to other avenues, like positive psychology and spiritual texts. My readings ranged from Wayne Dyer's *Real Magic* to the *Vedanta*, a Hindu philosophical treatise. This was controversial ground for an agnostic, but here is where I found faint inklings of an answer. Being brought up in a Hindu tradition, it was easy to accept the philosophical underpinnings of the *Vedanta,* which read more like a book of science rather than a religious text, insisting on internal observation and experimentation as a means to knowledge. I also read Christian science, which had striking similarities to the Hindu philosophy; both emphasised that consciousness was all important, embodied in the phrase "I am," while material reality was transient and illusory, termed "Maya". This was in stark contrast to conventional scientific viewpoints, but had a lot of similarity with quantum physics, which proves the validity of 'hard to believe' theories like matter and energy are interchangeable states and the relativity of time and space.

I was fortunate to have been attuned to Reiki healing by a medical doctor during this time, which opened up a wealth of synchronicities in my life. Reiki is a hands-on energy healing system in which a practitioner channels universal energy through their hands to the recipient's body to heal various issues. Reiki, I discovered, healed on many different levels, not just physical. By becoming in tune with our "chakras," or centres of energy, through Reiki, one can learn to do incredible things. Through Reiki attunement, I actually found a way to manifest reality.

I will mention a couple of synchronicities which powerfully shaped my beliefs during this time. It was Consciousness's way of inviting me into its arms.

At the end of internship, we were eligible to sit for postgraduate entrance examinations to get into a specialty of our choice. By this time, I had firmly made my decision to specialise in psychiatry. My experiences so far had taught me that medicine was still largely mechanistic and functioning within those limited walls baulked the wanderer within me. I thought that my strong desire to connect with people as human beings rather than machines to be fixed by science would be more aligned with the field of psychiatry. Although not a popular choice conventionally, toward the end of my internship the demand had rapidly gone up, and thus I would require quite a high rank to get into the training program of my choice. I did my research and found that I needed an exam rank in the top 70 to safely get into psychiatry. Now, I will be the first to admit that I was neither the brightest, nor the most hardworking student of my class. Considering the fact that over 4000 doctors would be sitting the exam, some of whom had been preparing dedicatedly for the entire year or more, the prospect was quite daunting.

Using the principles of Reiki and creative visualisation, I immersed myself in the belief that I *would* secure a rank within the first 70, and spent considerable time visualising this goal.

Lo and behold, on the day of the result, my ranking was 68! I found myself getting goosebumps all over. It had *worked.* I later found that a lot of my classmates who were smarter and worked harder than me did not get through, and although I was disappointed for them, my heart filled with gratitude for this miracle in my life. I can only attribute such accurate results to the specific intent that I used in my visualisation daily.

The next challenge came a few weeks later. I was dreaming of the perfect residency and career in psychiatry when the news came that the particular program I was interested in was being scrapped due to lack of adequate faculty. I cried my heart out the first few days, moping around the house. My mother, always the practical one, suggested that I take medicine instead, being a 'safe' choice. Yet I could not see myself as a mechanic, fixing people's bodies with one-size-fits-all pills only after the damage is done.

I came to a decision- I would rather drop the year and try the next year for the same program when it was back on again. I pity my poor family, who definitely must have thought I was loopy to do this! Yet they supported me, as they always do when I am intent on a vision. For a month I sought divine guidance by visualizing with great precision being able to continue the course. The next month, I was informed that the program had recruited new faculty and would not be scrapped!

Was this divine intervention, or my intention creating reality?

Well, I ask you: is there a difference?

I struggled with reconciling the validity of my internal experiences with the public's view, and I hesitated to tell many people about my experience with Reiki, anticipating that I would be derided about my interest in "spiritual mumbo-jumbo" and perhaps even pitied for my gullibility. For several years, I led a double life, pursuing body-oriented conventional medicine on one level, while secretly pursuing my passion of Mind-Body Medicine and alternative healing on the other, hoping to one day reconcile the two worldviews.

I started my residency in psychiatry full of hopes and dreams of working at the cutting edge of science. Surely psychiatrists would be very open to new and challenging ideas, being an emerging field at the frontier of science! Here again, I was in for a rude shock. The psychiatric community, I found, was even more conservative than the rest of medicine. In fact, having no objective diagnostic instruments yet, it behaved more like a religious body, with the DSM as its bible, purported as the truth, whereas in fact, it was nothing but a set of diagnostic criteria arrived at by consensus.

Sound familiar?

Even more concerning to me was the extent to which Big Pharma was involved in influencing clinical decisions. Most of the research that psychiatrists based their decisions on were funded by pharmaceutical companies which had a vested interest promoting their own products. This was not an environment where scientific curiosity could grow. For years I tried to conform, while at the same time seeking better and more effective ways to help people.

I finally found the courage to free myself from the need to conform when I left my regular nine-to-five job and ventured out on my own terms a couple years ago. I had decided to open my own practice. What an incredibly frightening, yet liberating decision it was! Since then, I have noticed an exponential growth in my knowledge and my ability to help others. The process has been like piecing together an enormous jigsaw puzzle—and I am the first to admit that large chunks of the puzzle still are missing, or maybe even incorrect. But that is the beauty of science and even life. It is a constant journey of discovery and rediscovery, a never-ending source of mystery for our never-ending curiosity.

It has taken me two decades to let go of the veil of secrecy I have maintained and declare that I am a quantum psychiatrist—one who embraces the mysteries of the universe and tries many new, creative solutions (not just the one other doctors or Big Pharma suggest) to find the best help for my clients. To embrace this, I have had to let go of fear of public opinion or conformity and pursue a spirit of scientific curiosity, finding the truth not just by external observation, but also through direct experience.

I now have access to a range of diagnostic and treatment methods with which I am able to heal mental illnesses on different levels. Quantum psychiatry goes beyond medications or talk therapy, and many clients who were previously considered "treatment -resistant" have benefited from the lesser known interventions in my practice. By writing this book, I hope to spread awareness about these interventions that could potentially benefit many more people in the years to come.

Part I

THE THEORIES SHAPING QUANTUM PSYCHIATRY

Chapter 1

TINKER, TAILOR, SOLDIER, SAILOR

"The world as we have created it is a process of our thinking. It cannot be changed without changing our thinking."

—Albert Einstein

Why is Psychiatry everybody's business?

Mental illness is all around us. Chances are that everyone either suffers from, or has a family member or friend or close acquaintance who suffers from a mental illness. So it is everyone's business to know what a psychiatrist is.

The definition of a psychiatrist in the Oxford Languages dictionary is a "medical practitioner who specialises in the prevention, diagnosis, and treatment of mental illness."

Pretty straightforward, huh? That's until you look up the definition of mental illness in the same dictionary: "a health condition involving changes in thinking, emotion, or behaviour." When you consider that thinking, emotions, and behaviour are the main ways that we experience the world and the world experiences us, the ubiquitousness of the problem becomes evident.

The gamut of mental illness can include conditions ranging from intellectual disabilities, psychoses, depression, and traumatic experiences, to subtler conditions like dissatisfaction, interpersonal dilemmas, and relationship issues, to grief, bereavement, and even existential issues. This enormous scope is perhaps why anti-psychiatrists crusade to end the medicalization of social problems.

Yet, in truth, where do you draw the line between what is behavioural, what is emotional, and what is social? An attempt to cater to differing theoretical schools resulted in the current atheoretical classification. There is an interesting parable about six blind men who were asked to describe an elephant. One person felt the trunk and described it as a snake, another one felt a leg and described it like a tree, the third person felt its tail and described it as a rope, and so forth. Unfortunately, mental illness can often be like the proverbial elephant. Our current classification system shies away from explaining the cause of illness and prefers just to describe and treat what we are aware of, like we are the six blind men.

Herein lies the scientific paradox: how can you treat something if you don't know what it is or what causes it?

Conventionally, diagnosis is based on a clinical interview and the expectation is for the mental condition to neatly fit into a particular category in the classificatory system. Thereafter, we treat this condition either with medication or psychotherapy, or both. Unfortunately, mental illnesses are not well behaved creatures and they refuse to fall into neat categories, much to the frustration of us psychiatrists! Even those who do fall into these categories refuse to respond predictably to treatment. Patients often spend years searching for the elusive happy pill or the perfect therapy which will help solve their problems, never finding just the right solution.

A man who had lost his wife a few years ago and is struggling to find meaning in life is treated with the same pills as a man who is unhappy with his job but feels trapped in it due to financial reasons. A woman who has endured unspeakable childhood abuse undergoes the same cognitive behavioural therapy as a woman going through a marriage breakdown. We try our best to individualise therapy, but this is impossible with the limited therapeutic repertoire that we currently base our practice on.

Yes, you heard me right. Our current official therapeutic repertoire is limited, despite all the new drugs on the market (which are variations of the old), and the new therapies (which are largely adaptations of the old). The key word here is "official". In future chapters, I will be talking about diagnostic techniques and treatment interventions that exist today, yet do not feature in any psychiatric textbooks or standard psychiatric literature. Despite that, they are promising and just might be the future of psychiatry—if we overcome our prejudice and allow them into the mainstream. The challenge we face today is not so much if effective treatments exist, but if we are willing to let go of our current worldview and take a quantum leap.

Why is Quantum Psychiatry everybody's business?

Psychiatry today, despite what people might think, is largely a mechanistic discipline focusing on the brain and its chemical milieu. Many of the psychiatric theories focus on brain neurotransmitters (chemicals released by nerve endings that transmit information across the brain) and how their deficiency or excess causes mental illness. For example, low serotonin levels are found in people who have depression, so therefore restoring the level of serotonin at certain nerve endings can help relieve symptoms of depression. This forms the basis of treatment with medications such as antidepressants, mood stabilizers, and antipsychotics.

On the other hand, *psychology* focuses on the mind and has a variety of views and approaches. Psychology today is very fragmented. It can be intensely political as well, as people can identify with a particular school of thought and disregard other schools. Behaviourists have a here-and-now approach, focusing on current thoughts and behaviours, while analytical psychology focuses on how past experiences shape present thought and behaviour.

Also we have humanistic psychology, focusing on the self, and more recently positive psychology and energy psychology, with a focus on vital energy as the instrument of change. It is evident to the discerning mind that the fields of psychiatry and psychology pose at least two challenges.

Firstly, inherent in the current model is the concept of mind-body dualism, which was first proposed by Rene Descartes, a 17th century French philosopher and scientist. The brain is seen as matter and is treated with chemicals, which are also matter, to orchestrate a change in the "mind", in the form of improved thoughts. Similarly, various psychotherapies, which work on the mind, eventually have an effect on the brain, as demonstrated by restoration in the level of neurotransmitters and size of some key brain regions that shrink in depression. Yet no one has been able to find that elusive step where matter (brain chemicals) is transformed into thought. This is almost considered taboo, because the moment we look this paradox in its face, our current Newtonian (mechanistic) approach falls apart.

Secondly, and perhaps as a result of our assumption that mind and brain are separate, the field of psychiatry is very fragmented. As with any other fragmented field, emotions run deeper than science. As aforementioned, psychologists identify themselves by the school they belong to— "I am a cognitive behaviourist" or "I am a psychoanalyst" they say— and vehemently defend their school of theory. The picture is similar with psychiatrists. There are experts on bipolar disorder, who categorise this illness into seven subtypes (while others only recognise one or two types). Some psychiatrists tend to diagnose ADHD very often, while others deny even its existence! And so the list goes on. Yet, science does not need defenders. Science is observable and replicable and does not need a "father figure". Hence the need for a unified theory that will be observable, replicable, and not need defending.

While psychiatry is the study of mental illness, psychology is the science of consciousness. Thus psychology is a broad field studying all human experiences, positive and negative, while psychiatry is more exclusive to disordered experience. Yet, one cannot exist without the other. Thus in my discussions, you will often find that I intertwine psychology and psychiatry—not deliberately, but simply because separating them would be like taking the two helices of a DNA strand apart. It's possible, but without meaning or purpose.

The basis of quantum psychiatry is quantum physics, which states that consciousness, or the observer, is the primary instrument of experience. In other words, in quantum psychiatry we move away from the assumption that the brain is the seat of consciousness but rather, the reverse is true: the brain is a manifestation of consciousness. This concept can be hard to wrap your head around, but quantum physics seems to read like a plot out of Alice in Wonderland! Consciousness, as quantum physicist Amit Goswami points out in *The Everything Answer Book*, is inclusive of the brain, experiences of the mind, vital experiences, intuitive experiences, and experiences of self. A more detailed explanation will follow in section one.

Quantum psychiatry is an attempt to develop an all-inclusive model of mental health and illness on all these layers of existence of consciousness. It is a practical application of the principles of quantum physics to understand the maladies of the mind-brain-body and treat it according to the same principles. Quantum psychiatry will address the gaps and paradoxes in our current knowledge.

This Book

In this book, I hope to share with you the importance of acknowledging our multi-dimensional existence, without which treatment of mental illness is limited.

If you or someone you know or love is suffering from a mental illness, I hope that this book will open your mind to this new paradigm in psychiatry which holds a lot of promise and the potential to heal on many different levels. If you are reading this book out of scientific curiosity, I hope to engage you not just in a scientific discussion but also encourage you to do your own research, as I have done, to arrive at your own conclusions. Quantum psychiatry, like quantum physics, is as ancient as the scriptures and as new as the particle accelerators. It belongs to no one and everyone. It is evidence-based and I hope it will unify the fields of psychiatry and psychology in the near future.

This book is divided into three sections. **Section One** explores some basic theories of quantum physics as they relate to the brain-mind and forms the basis of the next section. **Section Two** describes the application of quantum theory to psychiatry and the various diagnostic and interventional modalities available to our multilayered existence. **Section Three** is a series of meditations designed to help you experience some of the concepts outlined in section one. These meditations are leveled, so you are able to go deeper and deeper into quantum consciousness progressively.

Each section of the book can be read on its own. Section One is for the scientifically oriented and the sceptics. Here, I discuss the framework on which quantum psychiatry is built and provide a lot of theory and evidence. If you find this part too information-dense, feel free to jump to Section Two, which takes you through a range of practical therapeutic interventions along with some of my personal experiences with myself or clients. Section 3 and the appendix are mainly experiential; the meditations can be read on their own, but will be more meaningful if you have read both parts before. The meditations are also available in mp3 format to download on my website 'www.thequantumpsychiatrist.com', so that you can listen to and practice them regularly.

A word about the clinical examples: Most of them are drawn from my own clinical practice, however, I have changed names, ages and details of history significantly to preserve their anonymity.

So, I invite you to take a journey with me into the multilayered human consciousness and delve into its disorders and multiple modalities of treatment. Are you ready to take a quantum leap?

Chapter 2

ADVENTURES IN WONDERLAND

QUANTUM PHYSICS AND THE BRAIN

Concerning matter, we have been all wrong.
What we have called matter is energy, whose vibration
has been so lowered as to be perceptible to the senses.
There is no matter. There is only light and sound."

—Albert Einstein

What separates us humans from other life forms is the fact that we question who we are from the moment we are able to think. We are fascinated by the question- What makes us tick?

We are both the clock and the mechanic, as we try to pry open our brains to see how they work. We have made amazing progress into knowing a lot about the brain—its anatomy, cellular structure, physiology—and we are now even able to observe it working in real-time, through technological advancement. 1990-1999 was declared the Decade of the Brain by U.S. President George Bush, as more and more funds were pumped into brain research. Fast forward thirty years and we still cannot confidently say that we know how the brain and consciousness work. Biologist Lyall Watson calls this the "Catch 22" of the biology of consciousness: "If the human brain were so simple that we could understand it, we would be so simple that we couldn't" (Brain Mind Bulletin, 1979, p.3)

One of the most vexing questions for scientists is the question of how matter can transform into thought. We might know all about how neurons fire and transmit signals to induce a variety of neurotransmitters, and we may be aware of correlations between different brain regions or neurotransmitters with mental disorders, yet the fundamental question remains: How does a neuron firing or a neurotransmitter produce thought?

In fact, we don't even know the answer to the question: "What is thought? Where does it arise and where does it go?"

Cartesian duality has only widened the divide between the brain and mind to the extent that we hesitate to even discuss the linking step between the two.

Interestingly, there is only one theoretical field that can dare to answer these questions: quantum physics. A true understanding of quantum physics is so mind-boggling that it dissolves the very world we live in. For the reader who is not familiar with the concepts of quantum physics, I will refer them to read *The Self Aware Universe* by Amit Goswami. I will be discussing a few basics here, but a more detailed discussion is beyond the scope of this book.

Quantum simply means "packets". Different kinds of energy exhibit properties of both waves and particles. This is demonstrated by the double slit experiment, in which light passing through two slits is observed on a screen behind the plate. The wave nature of light causes the waves to interfere and produce dark and bright bands on the screen. However the light is absorbed at the screen at discrete points, demonstrating that light is also a particle. Since matter is nothing but slowed down energy, all objects are quantum in nature, with both wave and particle qualities. However, these waves are in fact "waves of possibility," since Heisenberg, a German physicist, in his famous uncertainty principle, proved that it is not possible to measure the velocity and position of a particle simultaneously with any certainty. The actual particle is likely to be found where the undulations of the wave are greatest, but this is a probability, rather than a certainty. Thus an electron within an atom can be simultaneously at various different positions at the same time. However, when an observer witnesses the electron, it is found in a particular location, a phenomenon called "collapse". Thus all phenomena remain in the realm of possibility unless an observer, who is non-material, is involved. John Von Neumann, a brilliant mathematician, in his 1932 book *The Mathematical Foundations of Quantum Physics,* proved that no material interaction is capable of converting waves of possibility into actuality. It is the observer, or what we call consciousness, that collapses the waves of possibility into actuality. Thus, what we call "reality" only exists because we are the observers.

Whereas neuroscience assumes that the brain is the seat of consciousness, quantum physics infers that consciousness is the ground of all being and thus it is not a brain phenomenon. The neuroscientific approach, where we are nothing but matter, creates a paradox. Matter can be broken down into smaller and smaller fractions until we are left with infinitesimally small particles, but this still cannot create the subjectivity that is a part of existence: the sense of "I" ness.

Dr. Amit Goswami, noted theoretical physicist and former professor of quantum physics at the University of Oregon, explains this materialistic viewpoint as the old school of upward causation, whereby we assume that elementary particles build atoms, which build molecules, then cells, which make up the brain, and the brain causes consciousness.

Quantum physics, on the other hand, postulates that consciousness, or the observer, is "primary" (comes before the brain or anything else), thus there is downward causation: consciousness causes all material interactions. Consciousness chooses one facet out of many facets, which becomes actualised into material reality. This is the same phenomenon as with the waves of possibility: "collapse". Consciousness is all-pervasive and not necessarily localised to the brain.

Why then, do we identify with our brain and not see it as an organ separate from "us"? Dr. Goswami introduces the concept of "Tangled Hierarchy" to address this question. In simple hierarchy, a lower level affects a higher level. In tangled hierarchy, the levels of causality are so intertwined that it is not possible to determine which is the lower level and which is the higher. Thus we identify with the images of external objects reflected on our brains and become one with them, creating the impression that the brain is our seat of consciousness. The observer is the observed.

The next vexing question that quantum physics can answer is the nature of thoughts, feelings, and intuition. As we have seen before, it is not possible to break down matter into its smallest particle to get a thought, feeling, or intuition. Thoughts, feelings, and intuition are waves of quantum possibility in consciousness, which are represented in the physical (i.e. our brains and bodies).

In his book *The Emperor's New Mind*, mathematician Roger Penrose noted that matter cannot process "meaning", as simple algorithmic computations cannot lead to meaning. Consciousness is required to produce meaning. According to Goswami in *The Quantum Doctor*, in the last century, quantum physics has recognised what ancient civilizations knew intuitively. Human beings exist at different levels of consciousness with physical, vital or energetic, emotional, mental, and supramental levels, a concept known as psychophysical parallelism. The vital or energetic level is a holographic image of the physical body, which extends beyond the physical body. The emotional body, as the name implies, consists of our feeling states. The mental level is the level of our thoughts, while the Supramental level consists of our intuition and creativity. These layers envelop the physical body, much like a set of nested Russian dolls.

Mainstream medicine is usually concerned with upward causation. Thus, it uses lower levels of the body to influence higher levels. For example, an antidepressant increases the level of serotonin in the brain (physical) which in turn affects our emotions and thoughts (emotional and mental layers). On the other hand, many alternative systems of healing follow a path of downward causation. For instance, hands-on energy healing systems like Reiki influence the vital and mental bodies, which then heal the physical body. Once we understand this model, it is easy to see how, although different, both are valid approaches.

Chapter 3

SPOOKY ACTION AT A DISTANCE

SIGNAL-LESS COMMUNICATION

"Nothing happens until something moves. When something vibrates, the electrons of the entire universe resonate with it. Everything is connected."

—Albert Einstein

In the world of quantum physics, everything exists in the domain of pure potentiality, beyond our ordinary concept of time and space. In the domain of pure potentiality, communication does not require a medium and is not dependent on the distance between objects. When two objects are in a state of correlation, also called quantum entanglement, communication between them is instantaneous, regardless of the distance between them. Einstein, Podolsky, and Rosen, they proposed in a famous thought experiment that when two particles are entangled, changing the spin of one of the particles would instantaneously change the spin of the other particle in the opposite direction, regardless of the distance between them. This essentially created a paradox, as it meant that communication could take place at a speed faster than the speed of light, which is forbidden by the theory of relativity. However, it is not really a contradiction, as only communication through space and time is limited to the speed of light, while signal-less communication occurs in the field of potentiality, or "the unmanifest".

Signal-less communication has long been known to exist in spiritual traditions, but until the last century, science had been unable to prove it. Quantum entanglement can now explain phenomena like distance healing, telepathy and other psychic phenomena which are based on the ability to communicate instantaneously over long distances. Physicist Amit Goswami conducted an experiment to demonstrate that entanglement affects people. He had two people meditate together, and then meditate separately in two chambers where they could not see or hear each other. When a light strobe stimulated one of the meditators, it caused a firing of a particular frequency in their brain. At the same moment, the other meditator's brain also fired the same frequency, even though he was not exposed to the light. This is the principle of distance healing: the healer and healee are entangled, and communication is instantaneous.

I am well aware that a lot of "scientific" magazines disregard that quantum entanglement could be linked to distance healing and devalue energy healing, calling it nothing but "snake oil." However, these naysayers also do not seem to offer any scientific evidence to the contrary. As I said, science does not need detractors and defenders. All I ask the reader to do is to look at the evidence dispassionately and experience phenomena like energy healing for themselves to arrive at their own conclusion.

Chapter 4

THE GUARD DOG, THE ELEPHANT AND THE WISE OWL

THE NEUROSCIENCE OF MENTAL ILLNESS

"Everything should be as simple as it can be, but not simpler."

—Albert Einstein

If you are anything like me, you might be struggling with a lot of the concepts mentioned in the previous chapters. I hope I have made it brief and simple enough to hold your attention, but not too simple to render it meaningless. If you are feeling a bit dizzy in the head, like Alice after she went down the rabbit hole, don't be hard on yourself, you are in hallowed company. Neils Bohr, a Danish physicist and one of the fathers of quantum physics, once said "If quantum mechanics hasn't profoundly shocked you, you haven't understood it yet."

Now that we have had a dash of quantum physics to whet our palates, how about a sprinkling of neuroscience to tempt our tastebuds? If you have survived this far, the next few pages are going to be cakewalk!

What is the relationship between the brain and consciousness? We can compare consciousness to a wireless signal while the brain is a receiver. Now, if you are unable to load the Google homepage on your phone, there might be several causes—for instance, you might be disconnected from the Wi-Fi network, or the phone itself might be broken. In both cases, there will be no internet access. Similarly, while consciousness is important, the brain needs to be working correctly in order to receive the right information.

Most of us know from school biology lessons about neurons, which are the basic cells of the brain carrying electrical signals across various pathways. The space between two neurons is called a synapse. Certain chemicals in the brain, called neurotransmitters, mediate communication between different neurons across the synapse. Although there are many different neurotransmitters, the commonest you will hear about in psychiatric parlance are serotonin, norepinephrine and dopamine. Simplistically speaking, serotonin regulates mood, norepinephrine regulates mood and arousal, while dopamine is involved in cognition and attention. Imbalances in these neurotransmitters have long been thought to be the basis of many mental illnesses, like depression, anxiety, schizophrenia, addictions, and ADHD—though now, through quantum psychiatry, I know the truth is often more complex than it may appear.

Riding the brain waves

True to its quantum nature, the brain exists as both matter and energy. Signals are mediated through neurotransmitters, and these signals together produce brain waves. These waves can be detected on the scalp using a technique called electroencephalography (EEG), whereby sensors attached to the scalp pick up brain activity which is translated into a graphical display.

There are five principal types of brain waves generated by the neurons: delta, theta, alpha, beta and gamma, named according to their frequency, measured in cycles per second, also known as hertz (Hz). They are akin to musical notes- some are low frequency and some are high frequency, and like an orchestra, they work together to produce a symphony in the brain.

Delta waves, ranging from 1-4 Hz, are found in deep sleep and are associated with restoring body and mind, while Theta waves (4-8 Hz) occur in dreamy and deep states like meditation. Alpha waves (8-12 Hz) are usually present in a state of relaxed awareness and is the resting state of the brain, while beta waves (12- 20 Hz) signify attention and focused mental activity. Another band of beta, called high beta (20-40 Hz) is usually associated with high anxiety, while gamma waves (>40 Hz), are related to higher level information processing and higher states of consciousness. None of the brain waves are good or bad, but it is the total combination that tells us if the symphony is well coordinated or discordant.

Why is it important to know about brain waves? Armed with this knowledge, you can learn to direct your orchestra to produce a glorious symphony, like a master conductor. Although brain waves are usually unconsciously produced, new technology now enables us to bring them under conscious control, so we can determine if the orchestra plays Beethoven's symphony, hip-hop music, or hard metal.

The animals in our brains

Our brains are divided into the hindbrain, midbrain, and forebrain, according to their location and development. The hindbrain, consisting of the cerebellum and brainstem, deals mainly with unconscious physiological processes, like breathing and respiration, amongst others, and is the first to develop. The midbrain consists of structures which form the limbic system, the emotional part of the brain, and develops next. The last to develop is the forebrain, or the cerebrum, the seat of our reasoning and judgement. The fact that the limbic system develops before the cerebrum, is the reason why we often find that our emotions and impulses "kick in" before we have a chance to think the situation through. How does this happen? And how can we control it?

A couple years ago, my daughter, who had just started school, was regularly having meltdowns at home. I was at my wit's end, feeling helpless despite my many years of training and experience in the field. It was then that I discovered an easy and interesting way to explain the neuroscience of emotions to a five-year-old (and anybody): Let's talk to the animals in our brain.

Deep in the limbic system is a structure called the amygdala, which regulates fear responses and is vital to the pathogenesis of psychiatric illnesses. The amygdala is the guard dog in the brain. When things are going on as usual, the guard dog sleeps. Let us imagine that you are walking in a park when you suddenly spot a four-legged, furry, brown creature bounding towards you. The guard dog is alert at once and sends information to the hippocampus—or the memory centre, the elephant in the brain. The elephant goes through its memories and recalls that a similar creature, which it identifies as a dog, had once bitten you when you were younger and you had to go to the hospital. It relays this information back to the guard dog. Now, the guard dog is upright and snarling away at the threat, which the elephant just informed him is real. *Voila*, you are in a "fight or flight", or panic mode. The only animal that can calm the guard dog is the wise owl, the neocortex—otherwise known as the brain's seat of judgement. The wise owl tells the guard dog that the previous time it had happened, the dog was not on a leash and was ferocious, while this one is with his owner and is friendly. However, there is a catch—the guard dog is getting bigger and more ferocious with every second, and if the wise owl is too late, the guard dog is out of control.

People who have had previous traumatic experiences have a guard dog that is perpetually aroused and never sleeps. Thus, even seemingly innocuous stimuli can trigger a panic attack. The wise owl is not strong enough to be heard by the guard dog, which practically rules the show.

We can see most psychological treatments as intervening on one of the animals. Cognitive therapy focuses on strengthening the wise owl, while mindfulness helps to keep the wise owl in the present moment. Yet newer techniques like limbic therapy specifically work on calming the amygdala, and therapies like eye movement desensitization and reprocessing (EMDR) target the elephant and helps process negative memories.

Although I run the risk of oversimplification, I find this framework very helpful to explain many mental illnesses like anxiety, panic disorder, and post-traumatic stress disorder. This model also gives a common language to engage our intellect when emotions run high. When I explained the animals to my daughter, not only did she have loads of fun imagining all the animals running around merrily in her brain, but it was also easy for me to say to her in the middle of a temper tantrum, "Where is your wise owl?" or, "Don't let your guard dog wake up!" to stop a meltdown from happening. A few months later, I found her literally "talking to her brain" with statements like, "Think, wise owl!" and "Remember, elephant!"

Top down, bottom up, or both ways?

As you might have noticed, communication within the limbic system is bidirectional, with the limbic system informing the cortex and vice versa. A healthy limbic system preserves this flow of communication, while disruption to the normal flow results in illness. Traditional talk therapy, whether psychodynamic, cognitive, or behavioural, is a top-down approach, mainly working on the neocortex. However, those whose amygdala are over aroused due to years of abuse or negative self-talk often report that although they know how to challenge their beliefs, they do not believe it in their heart. On the other hand, approaches like neurofeedback and EMDR are bottom-up, focusing on regulating the amygdala. For optimal results, a combination of top-down and bottom-up therapies are needed, especially for people with chronic and deep-seated issues.

Mirror, mirror in my brain

In the 1990s, Rizzolatti and colleagues at the University of Parma, Italy were studying the macaque monkey. They found that certain groups of neurons in the monkey's brain would fire when they picked up food. Interestingly, the same parts of the brain would fire when the monkey saw one of the researchers pick up food. These special neurons were named mirror neurons, and are found especially in the parts of the brain associated with motor actions and planning.

Mirror neurons have only been described in primates and songbirds and are believed to play an important role understanding the intention of another person doing an action. Mirror neurons help us develop a "theory of mind", whereby we are able to understand that others have thoughts and intentions separate from us. Scientists have proven that children with autism spectrum disorders have dysfunctions of the mirror neuron system, which makes it hard for them to relate to people. On the other hand, people who are more empathic have been shown to have stronger activations in both motor and emotional mirror neuron systems.

What I find particularly interesting is the role of mirror neurons in visualisation. Mirror neurons are activated when an individual is watching a set of motions to be learnt. Even more intriguing is the fact that visualisation activates these same neural networks as the actual physical activity! Elite sports athletes have used visualisation for decades to improve their performance and set records. There is ample research on the role of visualisation in cancer remissions. Visualisation is a powerful, but woefully underutilised tool for management of psychiatric disorders.

If this interests you, the guided meditations in Part 3 of the book use creative visualisation principles. The concept that "Thought directs matter" is embodied in the exercises, and their repeated practice will help strengthen the relationship between the thought and the goal.

Chapter 5

GLIA AND EINSTEIN'S BRAIN

"Imagination is more important than knowledge. For knowledge is limited, whereas imagination embraces the entire world, stimulating progress, giving birth to evolution."

—Albert Einstein

Since we are on a very interesting journey through our brains, having visited the orchestra and the animals within, let's now take a look into the Brain of the Century and see if it holds any more mysteries for us to decipher.

Albert Einstein is recognised as a genius and had perhaps the most fascinating mind of the 20th century. Because of his genius, scientists wondered if his brain was different from an average human brain. In 1985, scientist Marian Diamond found, disappointingly, that Einstein's brain did not contain more neurons overall than the average person's. It did, however, contain more astrocytes in the left inferior parietal area of the brain, the region associated with mathematical thinking. This finding was largely ignored at that time as astrocytes, a kind of glial cell, was only considered to be the "brain glue" that held neurons together. Only in the last decade has the role of glia been increasingly studied and recognised.

There are many types of glial cells, but the astrocytes are the most abundant cell in the human cortex. They extend their protoplasmic feet to blood vessels and neuronal synapses. Glia are the adult stem cells in the brain, meaning they can reproduce themselves and other neurons if needed—for example, after a stroke or injury. They can also regenerate locally to store more information. Interestingly, the ratio of glia to neurons increases with intelligence across species, as does the size of the glia, although we don't know the significance of this yet.

Recently, there has been more research into glial cells which have revealed some startling facts. Researchers have inserted human astrocytes into the brains of newborn mice and found that these mice became more intelligent. Their hearing and memory were also found to be sharper than other mice. Researchers have found that a synapse (the bridge between two neurons) is not just made of two neurons, but also an astrocyte. Astrocytes nurture synapses and they are the key to synaptic plasticity. One astrocyte can be in contact with as many as two million synapses, enabling coordination and communication across vast realms of the brain.

As early as 1966, Diamond demonstrated that rats, when put in a stimulating environment, had an increase in glial cells. This happens even in elderly mice. Plasticity takes energy and effort, and by nature our brains are lazy. They will only grow if given a good reason. Novelty or challenge gives the brain a reason to grow.

Recently, a study in 2016 revealed that insulin and leptin acts on astrocytes to regulate sugar intake in the brain. Lack of these receptors on astrocytes can lead to abnormal glucose metabolism and obesity.

In a study in 2019, researchers at the Advanced Science Research Centre, City College of New York, exposed test mice to an aggressive mouse for five minutes per day for ten days. They were then placed with an unfamiliar mouse to see if they showed signs of social withdrawal or were resilient. The mice who were socially withdrawn had fewer mature oligodendrocytes (a type of glial cell) and irregular myelin coverage (a sheath covering nerves) in the medial prefrontal cortex, a part of the limbic system or emotional brain.

It has also been hypothesised that lack of glial regeneration could lead to degenerative diseases like Alzheimer's dementia, while excessive regeneration leads to tumours. Gradually our understanding is changing as we realise that neurons only fire at the beck and call of glia to other glial areas to produce thought.

More recently, researchers are gathering evidence of the role of glia in psychiatric illnesses. While studying the post-mortem brains of the clinically depressed, researchers noticed the reduction in the number of astrocytes when compared with non-depressed brains. Astrocytes signal each other through intracellular calcium, which is postulated to be one of the pathogenetic mechanisms of bipolar disorder—too much produces mania, and too little causes depression. Reduced astrocytes have also been found in the brains of people with schizophrenia. In addition, even substances like cannabis and alcohol exert their effects through the calcium waves of astrocytes.

Such is the importance of glial cells that author and researcher Andrew Koob calls them "The Root of Thought". It is thus evident that glia are largely responsible for what we call "neuroplasticity"—or, should we say, "gliaplasticity"!

Previously, cognitive decline in ageing was thought to be the result of loss of neurons. However, interestingly, neuronal numbers seem to remain the same as we age. But there is something called an "astrocyte reaction" that happens in response to ageing, trauma and diseases of the brain. This probably explains why neural stem cell therapy has not really proven to be effective in degenerative disorders of the brain.

Recent research is focusing on using astrocytes to reverse brain disease.

Reading about astrocytes, one might wonder: How can one improve astrocyte functioning? Is there a way we can prevent degeneration from happening, or at least slow the progress? It seems disappointing that most glial interventions are only in the research stage and, so far, most research seems to focus on invasive treatments. However, there is a particular intervention which is believed to modulate astrocyte functioning non-invasively.

As I have discussed in the previous chapter outlining basic neuroscience, there are several types of brain waves: alpha, beta, theta, delta, and gamma. These are generated by neurons and are typically in the range of 1-60 Hz. Less well-known is the fact that there are some even *slower* brain waves below 0.1 Hz, down to millihertz. These are known as slow cortical potentials, which are generated by the calcium waves of the astrocytes. These slow cortical potentials are believed to regulate our body's ultradian rhythms, rhythms that happen several times a day, like sleep, appetite, hormone production, etc. As well as managing these rhythms, these waves manage phases of sleep and brain plasticity. Since astrocytes are so ubiquitous in our brain and have a role in many psychiatric disorders, it comes as no surprise that modulating these slow cortical potentials has a significant effect on improving the brain's ultradian rhythms with a positive effect on sleep, energy levels, attention, and concentration. Hopefully you now have an idea of the rapidity with which neuroscience is changing (perhaps we should even name it gliascience)! As we continue to unravel the mysteries of the human brain, body, and more, I want to give hope to readers that real progress is being made in the management of mental illnesses, and we have interventions with real potential available now or in the near future. Strange as these concepts might sound right now, they will soon be common knowledge and available to everyone.

Chapter 6

THE SEAT OF THE SOUL

THE PINEAL GLAND

"You can't use an old map to explore a new world."

—Albert Einstein

Nestled within the crevices in the centre of our brain is a tiny, pine cone-shaped gland called the pineal gland. Also called the "master" gland and the "third eye", we are yet to discover the mysteries of this gland in its entirety. The pineal gland has been revered through the ages as the spiritual centre in the brain, our connection to the divine. Descartes considered it the seat of the soul, but later, it was thought only to be a vestigial organ, with no significant role. However, as we discover more about this unassuming gland, we realise that it is in fact a master gland that helps us realise that we are more than just our physical bodies.

The pineal gland is known to contain rod-like cells which are sensitive to light. This is what gave it the name of the third eye. It is connected to a part of the brain called the suprachiasmatic nucleus and regulates the biological clock of the body. The pineal gland secretes melatonin in the absence of light, and serotonin when it is exposed to light, thus regulating the sleep-wake cycle. In the last few decades, we have learnt some of the qualities of melatonin which makes it one of the body's miracle hormones. Most of us are aware that we can use melatonin in conditions like jet lag, and it is helpful to regulate the sleep-wake cycle in individuals who do shift work.

Less well-known than its use as a sleep aid is the fact that melatonin is a powerful antioxidant, 200 times more powerful than vitamin E. Due to this, it has been found to have anti-ageing effects. Melatonin also regulates growth hormone release, as well as influencing the release of sex hormones. Thus, it plays a vital role in growth and reproduction. The pineal gland also regulates the immune responses of the body and plays an active role in the body's defence system and tumour suppression. Melatonin suppresses insulin secretion and reduces the levels of leptin, the hormone that encourages the body to store fat. Thus, it is important in regulating metabolism and weight gain. Melatonin also reduces the level of antidiuretic hormone and vasopressin, two pituitary hormones that regulate the body's water balance. All in all, it is a master gland which regulates the function of the pituitary gland and other hormones of the body.

In recent years, researchers have isolated certain metabolites of melatonin, most notably DMT, which is known to have psychedelic effects. Dr. Rick Strassman, a psychiatrist, calls DMT the "Spirit molecule" , as it produces near-death and mystical experiences. Although only very small quantities of DMT (inadequate amounts to cause such experiences) have been isolated from human pineal glands, scientists have been intrigued nonetheless by the presence of DMT in this gland and wonder if indeed the pineal gland is the "seat of the soul", as Descartes once proposed. This gland might mediate our connection to the spiritual world.

The pineal gland is composed mostly of pinealocytes (cells which secrete melatonin), astrocytes, and microglia. It also contains piezoelectric crystals. Piezoelectric crystals produce electricity in response to pressure. These are proposed to mediate many of the functions of the gland. Because of its highly vascular structure and high blood perfusion, this gland is also very susceptible to calcification. Till recently, calcification of the pineal gland was believed to be a normal physiological process with no significance. However, recent studies have found that pineal gland calcification is associated with lower melatonin production, poor quality of sleep, and increased ageing. Pineal gland calcification has also been seen in people with Alzheimer's disease and autoimmune disorders like multiple sclerosis.

Fluoride in tap water can increase calcification of the pineal gland. While it is unclear if calcification can be reversed, it can certainly be reduced by reducing the intake of fluoridated water, among other things.

The Pineal gland and mental illness

After centuries of veneration by ancient cultures, the pineal gland was relegated to the status of a vestigial organ in the 18th century (although some authors continued to believe that it was related to mental illness and treated subjects with mental deficiency with pineal extracts). There has been renewed interest in the relationship of the pineal gland and mental illness, which extends to more than just sleep disturbances.

Schizophrenia:

A recent review published last year compiled twenty-nine previous studies on pineal gland abnormalities in schizophrenia. The authors found that in most patients with schizophrenia, mean night plasma melatonin levels were lower than in healthy people. There is a higher prevalence of pineal gland calcification in schizophrenia, and the gland volume was usually smaller as well. These characteristics were not related to duration of illness, suggesting them to be primary and possibly genetic based. Melatonin treatment was found to lead to modest improvement in sleep quality, metabolic side effects of antipsychotics, and reduced movement disorders.

Mood disorders:

Most people with mood disorders, whether bipolar disorder or depression, have disturbances of their sleep-wake cycle. Bipolar disorder is closely linked to the body's biological clock and in fact, therapies for bipolar disorder focus on regulation of biological rhythms. However, a study comparing pineal gland volumes in schizophrenia, bipolar disorder, and depression (versus control groups) found significant reduction in volume in schizophrenia, but only small reduction in bipolar disorder and depression. Still, melatonin is widely used to manage insomnia in people with mood disorders.

ADHD: Recent research indicates that people with ADHD have a smaller pineal gland volume as compared to the normal population. Also, people with ADHD tend to have an evening circadian preference, which is hypothesised to be linked to the reduced volume. Sleep disturbances are very well known in people with ADHD and melatonin is commonly used to improve the circadian rhythm. However, it is uncertain if the smaller volume of the pineal gland is the result or the cause of poor sleep.

Alzheimer's dementia: It is now well documented that people who develop Alzheimer's dementia have high levels of calcification of their pineal gland and the volume of their gland is also decreased. This also correlated with low serum melatonin and disturbed sleep-wake cycle.

Thus, there is abundant evidence that a lot of psychiatric illnesses are associated with decreased volume and function of the pineal gland, a fact that has not received its due importance in psychiatric literature so far. Is melatonin replacement the solution? The honest answer is, "I don't know." While it makes sense to replace lost melatonin given its many health-enhancing properties, there is a risk that long-term melatonin supplementation can cause feedback inhibition of natural melatonin production (too much melatonin causes a reduction in its production to restore homeostasis), a phenomenon seen with a lot of the body's hormones. Our knowledge of the gland and its functions is still in its infancy, so we are not aware if artificial melatonin would suppress other functions of the gland. As far as research indicates, melatonin supplementation is safe in the short term, but there is inadequate information about its long-term effects.

Are there ways to naturally enhance the pineal gland's function and improve melatonin production? Blogs and websites are full of information on ways to decalcify the gland and improve its functioning. Most, however, are not backed by research, except low level laser therapy.

Low level laser therapy (LLLT), also known as photobiomodulation, might help increase melatonin production, according to several researchers. First studied in 2001, researchers in China have found that applying intranasal low level laser once a day for ten days increased melatonin production. Since then, this has been confirmed by several other researchers. The pineal gland sits in the base of the brain, directly above the nasal plates of the skull, which are in fact permeable to light. Near infrared light used in LLLT easily penetrates the nasal capillaries and nasal bones to stimulate the base of the brain.

One of the best known LLLT devices is Vielight, founded by Dr Lew Lim. Vielight has robust research to back its clinical application in a variety of conditions ranging from insomnia to dementia to performance enhancement.

We are just beginning to discover the importance of our pineal gland in every facet of our life. There is enough evidence to suggest that calcification can hinder a lot of the gland's functions, thus, reducing the chances of this happening by reducing fluoride intake would be a reasonable step to take towards improving our health.

Chapter 7

BALL OF LIGHT

THE HUMAN ENERGY FIELD

"It would be possible to describe everything scientifically, but it would make no sense; it would be without meaning, as if you described a Beethoven symphony as a variation of wave pressure."

—Albert Einstein

Although the concept of a human energy field has been around for centuries in ancient cultures like India, China, and Egypt, it was considered mere spiritual lore until recently. Western medicine focuses mainly on physiology and biochemistry. But the organism interacts with a number of energies—light, sound, electricity, magnetism, etc.—and current Western Medicine needs to expand its concept to the human energy field to progress to the next level. Western Medicine already measures these biofields through diagnostic procedures like sonograms, magnetic resonance imaging (MRI), electrocardiography (ECG), electroencephalogram (EEG), cranial tomography (CT)and positive emission tomography (PET) techniques. Many might not be familiar with these techniques, but they all use the body's electrical and magnetic activities to diagnose problems. Biophotonics is being used in medical diagnostics to tag single intracellular protein molecules, allowing us to track molecular functions in real-time with a high degree of accuracy. However, although we use quantum mechanical and energy concepts for diagnosis, conventional medicine reverts back to biochemistry for treatment.

The scientific study of these fields started with Harold Burr, a professor of Neurophysiology at Yale University, USA, who called it the Life Field. He measured smooth fields in healthy adults but wild electrical patterns in patients with schizophrenia. He found changes in the Life Field to occur before physical disease set in.

Robert Becker, MD, was a researcher in the Department of Orthopaedic Surgery in New York. He published a landmark book, "The Body Electric", in which he pointed out the existence of steady electric currents outside neurons, which are non-ionic in nature. These currents, which were considered dipolar, seemed to determine an organism's growth and development. It is a testament to his work that Becker was cited for a Nobel Prize.

In 1923, Russian researcher Alexander Gurwitsch found that living tissues emit photons in the visible spectrum. Most of our current knowledge of biophotons comes from the works of Dr. Fritz-Albert Popp, who has been researching biophotons since the 70s. He hypothesised that biological regulation in the body is governed by photons, which are stored primarily in the DNA and create a holographic field , informing cells of their relative position in the overall blueprint. The body emits a steady stream of biophotons, which can be captured on Kirlian and Gas-Discharge Visualisation (GDV) cameras and which give an indication of the health of the organism. A significant amount of the biophotons are emitted by the neural cells, and is correlated to neural and EEG activity as well as cerebral blood flow. When the brain is calm, reflected in alpha brainwave activity, the biophoton emissions are coherent, and fluctuations in the emission correlate to the fluctuations in alpha waves in the brain.

A scientist from the Massachusetts Institute of Technology, Dr. Claude Swanson, has given a convincing explanation of the science of the human energy field and energy healing. He cites the work of Dr. Nikolai Kozyrev, a Russian astrophysicist, who described an energy called torsion in the 1960s. Every particle, such as electrons, protons, and neutrons, has a spin. Every time a particle accelerates, it produces a twisting effect in space because of its spin. Swanson proposes that the torsion field outside the body is a copy of the biophoton field inside the body, produced from the spin of the biophotons. According to Dr. Swanson, the torsion field is strong outside the body and correcting the torsion field outside the body can change the pattern inside the body and bring about healing. This torsion field forms the blueprint for the body's growth. Torsion fields have three components: one which travels at the speed of light, one which travels backwards in time at the speed of light, and a third that travels at near-infinite speed. Swanson believes that these fields mediate long-distance healing.

British biologist Rupert Sheldrake, in his book *A New Science of Life* (1981), extended the concept of the energy field to the behavioural field. The 100th Monkey Theory, initially mentioned by Lyall Watson in his book *Lifetide*, proposed that when a critical number of individuals learn a new skill, this skill is transmitted non-locally to other individuals of a tribe. Sheldrake proposed the concept of Morphic fields, which could explain such non-local learning. According to him, Morphic fields are organising fields for animal and human behaviour, social and cultural systems, or mental activity. He describes Morphic resonance as a process whereby such self-organising systems inherit a memory from previous similar systems. This implies that memory need not be stored inside our brains, which can be likened more to TV antennae rather than storage discs. Thus each individual inherits a collective memory from members of the species.

Morphic resonance can explain not only how proteins organise into organisms, but also how organisms are greater than the sum of their parts. Sheldrake and other researchers have conducted several studies to demonstrate how it is easier to learn things which have been in existence for a while as compared to new themes. Morphic resonance might also explain why several individuals have come up with the same invention or theory at the same time.The concept of Morphic fields and Morphic resonance might sound familiar to those who are aware of the work of Carl Jung, a pioneering psychiatrist of the 19th century and a student of Freud. Jung proposed the existence of a collective unconscious, a set of memories and themes shared by all humanity. This is perhaps the reason why many cultures have developed similar myths and theories independent of each other. Within the collective unconscious, Jung proposed the existence of Archetypes, a model image or idea that is shared by all humanity. Archetypes are representations of abstract concepts which humanity shares, and these Archetypes are found everywhere in our art, culture, and literature. Examples of common archetypes are the mother, the hero, and the villain. Archetypes embody abstract concepts and ideals like truth, justice, and beauty. Archetypes represent our capacity for abstract thought as opposed to other beings, and form our rich internal psychic life.

The layers of the aura

The human energy field is not just a clump of energy sitting on top of our bodies. The subtle energy is understood to be organised into several layers, as evidenced by Kirlian photography and other visualization techniques. Just beyond the physical body lies the etheric or vital layer, which contains the organising information or template for the physical body. This is the energetic field containing the chakras and meridians, which we will discuss next. Many eastern- and energy-healing techniques act primarily on this level. As one progresses in energy work, one becomes acutely aware of the movement of energy along the spine and sensations like buzzing, tingling or heat over various parts of the body. With experience, you can even learn to feel this layer push against your palms as you move your hands towards somebody.

The next level is the emotional body, which contains our feelings. While some feelings are transient, others, especially if related to abuse, neglect, or negative life experiences, tend to persist in our emotional bodies. We can sometimes identify them as a sensation of tightness or closeness in a certain part of the body, which usually relates to the particular issue we are dealing with. For example, if you have issues asserting yourself, you might experience an uncomfortable sensation in the pit of your stomach, while if you have issues with anger, it can manifest as chest tightness. These energies need to be released before healing can progress.

When I first started working on my own emotional layer through energy work, it was like an uncontrollable flood of emotions was released, although I was not sad. I could only describe it as a gush of release of all the pent up emotions I had held within, and I suddenly felt lighter and more buoyant. I felt more energised every day, although I was sleeping less and eating less than before! This is not an uncommon experience for people who start energy work. As esoteric as it sounds, there is a definite science and technique to working on the emotional body which anyone can follow with dedication and persistence.

The mental level contains our thoughts and impulses. Although we identify our thoughts as being generated in the brain, evidence suggests that thoughts are in fact generated in the mental plane but we identify them as being in our brains due to the process of "tangled hierarchy" described in Chapter 2. Thoughts which are strong, persistent, and repetitive tend to be held in the mental body and take on a magnetic power, which in turn influences our experiences in life. The optimist sees the glass half full, while the pessimist sees the glass half empty. Two people in the same car accident might interpret things differently. While one driver says, "Thank God I am alive," the other one frets and fumes about the damage to his front fender!

Thoughts tend to have a cascading effect. Have you had days when you think you just got off on the wrong side of the bed? Well, one negative thought leads to another and becomes a self-fulfilling prophecy. Multiply this by years, sometimes a lifetime, and you can see the whirlpool of negativity that many people are sucked into. Negative thoughts can be very tenacious and difficult to get rid of. It requires great vigilance, along with a lot of self-compassion and persistence to get rid of these weeds in our garden.

The supramental (or spiritual) body is the house of our intuition and creativity. It is our connection with our higher self and higher realms. This plane is only accessible when the perturbation in the etheric, emotional, and mental bodies has settled down. It is like the rainbow which is only visible after the storm has passed. As human beings, it is rare for most of us to be in constant connection to our higher selves. Our access to this level might manifest as flashes of sudden insight, inspiration, or creativity, which leave us as suddenly as they come upon us.

There are famous examples of great scientists and inventors who got their inspiration through dreams or visions. Thomas Edison, inventor of the lightbulb, would often sleep with a coin in his hand. He would access the subconscious through dreams and inspirations, but if he drifted into deep sleep, the coin would fall and make a noise, waking him up, so he could retain those inspirations. Nikola Tesla, another great inventor, was famous for his vivid visions. He turned these visions into inventions which were lightyears ahead of his time. In dreams, we suspend our chronic emotional and mental chatter and allow inspiration to befall us. It is inspiration which has propelled humanity forward and allows us a greater understanding of our lives and our purpose in this world. Even those who are emotionally stable and highly successful can suffer from a sense of disconnection and lack of purpose until they tune into their connection with their higher selves.

Consciousness mediates between these levels of existence. Bringing our awareness into the various levels of our existence is the beginning of healing ourselves.

Chapter 8

ENERGY VORTICES OF THE BODY

THE CHAKRAS

"That which is impenetrable to us really exists. Behind the secrets of nature remains something subtle, intangible, and inexplicable. Veneration for this force beyond anything that we can comprehend is my religion."

—Albert Einstein

While in medical school, I became intrigued by the concept of chakras. I was raised in an environment where people were comfortable with such terminology, so was always familiar with the metaphysical concept, but my scientific temperament refused to acknowledge the validity of subtle energy and chakras until I had "proof". My first confirmation of the existence of subtle energy came during my Reiki initiation, when one of our teachers took Kirlian photographs of our fingertips before and after the attunements and made some very accurate interpretations of each student's physiological and mental states. I still have the photograph from over twenty years ago, as a reminder of the subtle energy within and around us.

As I continued to practice the energy techniques through the years, my awareness of subtle energies gradually increased. Initially I would experience tingling, buzzing, heat, or cold sensations during energy healing and meditation. Gradually, the experiences became more pervasive in my day-to-day life. Nowadays I feel a constant buzzing in my spine and entire body throughout the day. During meditations, I often feel a sense of pressure in the centre of my forehead, or burning or tingling on the forehead or the vertex of my head. These sensations are vastly different to an experience of headache and do, in fact, correspond to periods of intense inspiration and creativity.

Yet, for people who have not experienced subtle energy, the concept can be quite challenging. There continue to be demands for "objective evidence". Ancient civilizations emphasised internal observation as the path to knowledge, perhaps because we need to go beyond the five senses to observe the quantum world.

Fortunately, over the last few decades, innovative technological development has allowed us to gather more objective evidence of these subtle energies and the existence of chakras. One of the modern techniques which can be used to visualise energy fields is Gas Discharge Visualisation (GDV). Dr. Konstantin Kortokov of St. Petersburg State University has developed and refined the technique to observe the energy state of a body with the help of the Biowell GDV camera. When a scan is taken, an electrical field is used to stimulate emission of photons from the skin, which is captured by the camera and mapped to different organs and energy meridians of the body. The signal from a particular individual depends on a variety of internal factors, like the balance of the autonomic and hormonal systems, overall health state, and the balance of the person's chakras.

What are Chakras?

Hindu sages described the chakras as the energy centres of the bodies. There are seven major chakras and many other minor chakras are becoming known. These chakras correspond to the major organs or glands of the body and are each associated with a nerve plexus (a network of nerves). Table 1 shows the chakras with corresponding gland and nerve plexus and the role they are purported to play:

Table 1

Chakra	Gland	Nerve Plexus	Role
Crown	Pineal	Pineal plexus	Connection to spirituality
Third Eye	Pituitary	Pituitary plexus	Intuition, imagination, wisdom
Throat	Thyroid	Thyroid plexus	Communication, self-expression, truth
Heart	Thymus	Heart plexus	Love, joy, inner peace
Solar plexus	Pancreas	Solar plexus	Self-worth, self-confidence, identity
Sacral	Adrenals	Sacral plexus	Sense of abundance, well-being, sexuality
Root	Gonads, reproductive organs	Sacro-coccygeal	Survival issues, sense of security

Candace Pert, a neuroscientist, has demonstrated that these glands and nerve plexuses corresponding to each chakra are rich in neuropeptides, which she calls the "molecules of emotion". The neuropeptides found in the brain are found throughout the body, but higher concentrations are found in these chakra regions. The chakras are thus like mini-brains and, as per Pert, we are like a "segmented worm" with a separate brain for each body segment.

This challenges the western concept that the brain is the seat of our emotions. Emotions are experienced in our whole body, as you can surely vouch for—who has not experienced a warm, fuzzy, expanding feeling in the chest when you experience love for someone? Or the sickening nausea and butterflies in the tummy just before an exam or an important interview?

Interestingly, the chakras also correspond to the psychosocial stages of human development as proposed by psychologists Eric Ericson and Abraham Maslow. Ericson proposed eight stages of development, based on the conflicts to be resolved as one grows, while Maslow described a hierarchy of needs, starting from physiological and safety needs and moving on to love, self-esteem, and finally self-actualization. Whilst Erikson's model was from birth to old age, Maslow's model is useful for later stages of development. The model I propose below combines traditional psychosocial stages with the corresponding chakra development during the period.

Root Chakra: Trust vs. mistrust

From birth to twelve months of age, infants learn to trust adults whom they are dependent on for caregiving. This corresponds to the development of the root chakra, which forms the basis of our sense of security about the world.

Sacral Chakra: Autonomy vs. shame

As toddlers (one to three years) begin to explore the world and themselves, they learn to establish their independence. They become more curious and explore their sexual and excretory organs. This corresponds to the development of the sacral chakra, which gives us a sense of well-being and comfort in our own bodies.

Solar Plexus Chakra: Initiative vs. guilt, Industry vs. inferiority

Between the ages of three to six, children learn to initiate activities and assert themselves in their interaction with others. This is Erikson's phase of Initiative vs. guilt. In primary school, from six to twelve years of age, they begin to compare themselves to their peers and either develop a sense of pride in themselves and their achievements or feel inferior because they don't measure up. This stage is referred to as the stage of Industry vs. inferiority. Both these stages correspond to the development of the solar plexus, the seat of our power and self-esteem.

Heart Chakra: Identity vs. role confusion and Intimacy vs. isolation

In adolescence (twelve to eighteen years), children start to focus on relationships, rather than solely on themselves. Peer groups become very important and they start questioning their role in the world or purpose in life. This stage is referred to the stage of Identity vs. role confusion During early to mid-adulthood (twenty to forty years), individuals learn to give and receive love and develop intimate long-term relationships. A person negotiates the conflict of Intimacy vs. isolation. Both these stages correspond to the development of the heart chakra, when we start to focus away from self to friends, to partner, to family, to community, to country, and ultimately to the world. The development of the heart chakra spans the longest and is often the most difficult to negotiate. We instinctively call people who have been unsuccessful in a relationship as "heartbroken".

Yet, this is the period of development that offers most choice. We do not have control over how we were treated in childhood, but it is through the heart chakra that we develop the power to choose love over hate, forgiveness over revenge, acceptance over suffering. Ancient traditions consider the heart chakra as the integrator that merges the lower and higher chakras into a more wholesome experience.

Throat Chakra: Generativity vs. stagnation

During middle adulthood (forty to sixty years), the focus often shifts from individual achievements to contributing to the world and others, in a way that is personally meaningful. People find satisfaction in expressing what they have learnt and passing on their knowledge to others. This corresponds to the development of the throat chakra, when we finally "own our story", express our truth honestly, and let go of pretences and societal expectations.

Third Eye Chakra: Integrity vs. despair

From their mid-sixties to the end of life, individuals reflect on their lives and either feel a sense of integrity or a sense of regret or despair. This corresponds to the development of the third eye, a realisation of the bigger picture, something beyond "doing": simply "being".

Crown Chakra: Self Actualization

Ericson's theory ends here but the chakras move on to the crown chakra. The opening of this chakra more closely corresponds to Maslow's self-actualization or self-realization, where knowing pervades without learning and bliss is all there is. This is a stage that most of us only aspire to, or catch brief glimpses of during meditation.

It is important to understand that this is only an indicative and not an absolute model. While this is usually how people develop, the rate of maturation is different for all individuals. Whilst some people might be extremely spiritual and access their higher chakras at an early age, many others might only be able to negotiate the first few chakras in their entire lives.

But the chakras are not to be mistaken as only physical organs or even mini-brains, as they do have an energetic basis. Scientist Rupert Sheldrake first proposed the concept of morphogenetic fields in the 1980s. Morphogenetic fields are learning and organising fields within and around an organ which determine the development of the organ. For example, a cardiac field becomes the heart.

It is proposed that chakras act as energy transducers—in other words, they convert physical energy to subtle energy and vice versa. Another explanation is provided by theoretical physicist Dr. Amit Goswami. He explains that consciousness selects what will appear physically, choosing from one of many probabilities that live within the non-physical and non-local or morphogenetic fields. Consciousness "chooses", and chakras transduce from the non-physical field into reality.

How do Chakras relate to light and sound frequencies?

Each chakra is associated with a particular frequency, and each chakra becomes aroused in the presence of this frequency through a process called harmonic resonance. Harmonic resonance is a phenomenon when a standing wave frequency comes into contact with an object tuned to the same frequency, causing the object to vibrate at a level matching the generated frequency. The lowest frequency that an object vibrates at is known as the fundamental frequency, or first harmonic, and subsequent harmonics are multiples of this frequency. This gives us a clue to the link between sounds and colours and why they affect particular chakras. Both sound and light are waves and have bands which vibrate at particular frequencies. Light vibrates at a much higher frequency than sound, but can be a harmonic of a sound frequency. Sound researchers have now translated the colour associated with each chakra into specific sound frequencies and musical notes. The table below illustrates the light and sound frequencies associated with each chakra, which shows us clearly the harmonic relationship between light and sound:

Chakra	Colour	Light Wavelength	Sound Frequency	Note
Root	Red	430-480 THz	432 Hz	A
Sacral	Orange	480-510 THz	480 Hz	B
Solar Plexus	Yellow	510-540 THz	528 Hz	C
Heart	Green	540-580 THz	580 Hz	D
Throat	Blue	610- 670 THz	672 Hz	E
Third Eye	Indigo	670-750 THz	720 Hz	F
Crown	Violet	>750 THz	768 Hz	G

Using Colour and sound to heal chakras:

Colour therapy has its roots in ancient civilizations of Egypt, Greece, India, and China, but only recently gained scientific attention. Robert Gerard, a scientist in the 1950s used electroencephalograph (EEG) to prove that colours affect the body and mind. According to his studies, the colour red increased the amount of energy in the body, while blue relaxed the body. Coloured light has been used medically in a variety of conditions. Blue light has been used to treat neonatal jaundice for decades, and full spectrum light is now being used in the treatment of cancers, seasonal affective disorders, anorexia, bulimia nervosa, and alcohol dependence. Schauss worked on the tranquilizing effect of colours and found that pink colour reduces aggressive behaviour and violence. Blue light is now being used to reduce pain in arthritis, as well as healing injured tissue and lung conditions, while red light has been used in the treatment of some forms of cancer. Colour can also be used to heal particular chakra issues. Readers who are interested in a detailed account of chromotherapy can refer to a concise article by Azzemi and Raza cited at the end of the book.

Similarly, the science of sound therapy has been in existence for centuries. Buddhist chants, Tibetan singing bowls and prayer wheels, and Hindu mantras are just some examples of sound therapy which are now gaining scientific validation. I will direct the reader to the works of Jonathan Goldman, one of the pioneering researchers of sound therapy for a more comprehensive understanding of sound therapy in healing mental disorders.

Chapter 9

RIVERS OF ENERGY

THE NADIS AND MERIDIANS

"If at first the idea is not absurd, then there is no hope for it."

—Albert Einstein

I will not be doing justice to my readers if I do not take some time to explain a concept related to and as important as the chakras, but perhaps not as well known. These are the nadis, or energy meridians of the body, through which vital energy is proposed to flow according to traditional eastern medicine. Hindu scriptures refer to them as nadis, while Chinese medicine refers to them as meridians.

There has been considerable research into the Chinese science of acupuncture, where extremely fine needles are inserted into the meridian system to manipulate the flow of "chi", or vital energy. Despite several positive studies (especially in areas of infertility, immunity, and other chronic medical conditions), acupuncture is still considered to be "alternative", since until recently it was believed that the meridian system lacked an anatomical basis.

However, researchers have now validated the existence of a new body system called the primo vascular system (PVS), which corresponds to the meridians described in Chinese medicine. The system was initially described in the 1960's by Bong-Han Kim of North Korea, but did not gain attention till 2002, when its existence was confirmed by researchers in South Korea. Since then, it has been verified by several research groups across the world.

The primo vascular system pervades the subcutaneous tissues, organs, fascia, etc. and are thread-like structures which contain primo fluid. This fluid is rich in extranuclear DNA, RNA, mononucleotides, and amino acids, the building blocks of information within our body. Primo vessels show electrical activity and are believed to act as optic channels of biophoton emission, while the DNA in the fluid may act as a photon store. These biophotons are believed to play a key role in cell development and differentiation.

The discovery of the PVS is able to explain how vital energy (in the form of biophotons) travels through the body and can be externally manipulated by therapies like acupuncture and acupressure to encourage healing. The DNA-rich primo fluid obviously plays an important role in growth and regeneration of the body. While the PVS is still to be charted in its entirety, it appears that the age-old concept of "chi" or "prana" is flowing in meridians and influencing one's health. This is finally being validated through research.

Energy meridians (or nadis) are classified as major or minor, depending on their location, and there are striking similarities between the Chinese and the Indian systems. The Chinese "chi" is very similar to the Indian "prana", although there is more emphasis on the influence of breath on prana. Recent research on biophotons indicate that living tissues are constantly emitting a stream of biophotons, which are related to oxidative metabolism in the mitochondria and other reactions, which are in turn influenced by respiration.

Ancient Indian texts describe the main channels as those that hug the spinal column closely—the central column (the Sushmna), the left-sided channel that stimulates the right side of the brain (the Ida), and the right-sided channel that stimulates the left side of the brain (Pingala). The Ida is said to correspond to the feminine aspect, while the Pingala corresponds to the masculine aspect. The Chinese tradition names these yin (masculine) and yang (feminine). The Ida and

Pingala are activated through the flow of breath in the nostril, left for Ida and right for Pingala.

Interestingly, Western knowledge of brain lateralization and functioning also correspond to this concept of Ida and Pingala. The left hemisphere (which is stimulated by Pingala in Hindu literature), is typically associated with "masculine" functions like logical and analytical thought processes, reasoning, mathematics, and numerical skills, while the right hemisphere (which is stimulated by the Ida in Hindu literature) is associated with "feminine" functions like intuition, creativity, imagination, empathy, trust, and self-awareness. Although the concept of right-brained and left-brained individuals belongs to the realm of pop-psychology, lateralization (the tendency to employ one area of the brain more than another) is a genuine phenomenon.

Intriguingly, it is observed that individuals tend to breathe through one nostril about 85% of the time, and switch every four hours or so. Applying the concept of Ida stimulating the right side of the brain and Pingala the left, it implies that we solely access either the right or left brain during these periods of time.

The nadis can be activated through specific breathing techniques called pranayama. Although there are numerous pranayamas of varying difficulty levels, I will talk about a few which are simple, brief and have immense benefits for mind and body. Even five minutes of pranayama, done correctly, can leave you feeling refreshed, while regular practice has been proven to alleviate mild depression and anxiety and have positive neurocognitive effects. It is certainly a good technique for those who are restricted in their ability to exercise and energise the whole body, and I would recommend it for anyone with a mental health condition. I find a lot of people suffering from mental health conditions also have sleep apnoea, and pranayama, by increasing the oxygenation of the brain, can improve some of the consequences of sleep apnoea, as well.

An easy way to balance the breath in both nostrils is through Bhastrika, or bellows breathing, which involves forceful inspiration and expiration, which results in high oxygen levels through both nostrils and in the brain. It has been recommended for mental health conditions through the ages and is known to relieve symptoms of sleep apnoea.

A gentler method to balance the breath is alternate nostril breathing or nadi shodhana, in which we simply block one nostril with the thumb and another with a finger and breathe alternately through each nostril. This is an amazingly quick technique to calm the autonomic nervous system down in as little as five minutes.

It has been established that many individuals who have been unfortunate victims of childhood abuse and neglect have deficits in the right hemisphere functioning. Allan Schore, an American psychologist and researcher in neuropsychology, is a proponent of what he calls “right brain psychotherapy”. He describes how the emotional bond between an infant and its caregiver can physically affect brain development. He says that this communication between baby and caregiver is primarily right brain to right brain. Thus, health professionals who treat those who have suffered developmental trauma need to bring right-brained techniques focusing on empathy, affect regulation, and non-verbal communication. However, despite the best efforts of therapists, the right hemisphere of such individuals is often offline and they find it extremely difficult to be in a situation requiring trust and letting go of vigilance. Their autonomic nervous system kicks into hyperdrive the moment they enter the therapist’s office and think of letting go of control. In such situations, I find it helpful to instruct clients to breathe through their left nostril for five minutes. This often brings the right hemisphere online again and they report feeling calmer and more connected.

On the other hand, those with depression and a lack of energy can get a boost from practicing right nostril breathing, which can increase the activity of the sympathetic nervous system.

Research shows alternate nostril breathing has a great benefit on anxiety and depression. A study by Marshall et al in 2013 even showed improved performance in language measures in those with post-stroke aphasia after alternate-nostril breathing.

Another technique with great mental health benefits is Ujjayi breathing (otherwise known as "Ocean breath", because it sounds like ocean waves). In this technique, inhalation and exhalation is done while constricting the pharyngeal passage, creating an obstruction to air flow and thus producing a harsh sound like the waves upon the shore. There is a lot of research on Ujjayi breath in improving depression, anxiety and even preliminary studies on PTSD.

It is important to note that while these techniques sound simple, they should be learnt under the supervision of trained teachers initially, to get maximum benefits.

Now that we have some understanding of some of the guiding theories and principles behind quantum psychiatry, in the next section we will look into a variety of interventions focused on different layers of the human body.

Part 2

QUANTUM LEVELS OF HEALING

Chapter 10

THE PHYSICAL BODY

"It is in fact, nothing short of a miracle that the modern methods of instruction have not yet entirely strangled the holy curiosity of inquiry; for this delicate little plant, aside from stimulation, stands mainly in need of freedom. Without this it goes to wrack and ruin without fail."

—Albert Einstein

In the last century, there has been a steady focus on studying the brain and its various chemicals as the seat of mental illnesses. We are in an age when sophisticated brain imaging techniques allow us to look into the structure and functioning of the brain as it performs tasks. Two developments in the late 20th century were pivotal for psychiatry. First was the discovery of medications like chlorpromazine and imipramine which could improve symptoms of mental illness. This discovery led to a focus on manipulating neurotransmitters in the brain to treat these conditions. Second was the development of sophisticated brain imaging techniques, which meant that we could study how the brain changed in mental illness. Thus was born the chemical hypotheses for several mental illnesses, namely depression, anxiety, and schizophrenia, which is prevalent even today. It was elegant in its simplicity: a depletion of serotonin caused depression, and replenishing serotonin led to symptomatic improvement. Functional imaging was able to zone in on specific areas of hypo or hypermetabolism in particular illnesses and even structural differences in the brain of individuals with depression or schizophrenia as compared to the general population.

This is the domain in which psychiatry largely operates even today. Our knowledge of brain neurotransmitters and neuropeptides which influence our thoughts and emotions has grown by leaps and bounds. We have a large armamentarium of medications which target specific neurochemicals of the brain to treat a variety of mental conditions. It looks like we are in a golden age, with "a pill for every ill".

Undeniably, medications form a large part of a treatment plan for mental illnesses even to this day. Most mental conditions do respond, albeit variably, to pharmacotherapy. When an individual is in the throes of depression and unable to function, antidepressants can be a blessing—one which has saved many lives. The miracles of pharmacotherapy are most evident in what we regard as predominantly biological illnesses, like bipolar disorder and schizophrenia.

Yet, looking on from the inside, there are a number of vexing problems that we are unwilling to acknowledge. Firstly, some illnesses have not been so easy to explain away by neurochemical hypotheses alone. Even more vexing are mental illnesses which stem from the fabric of social life, like developmental trauma, abuse, post-traumatic stress, general unhappiness and dissatisfaction, grief, and existential issues. As a solution, anti-psychiatrists, a fringe group who believe that psychiatry does more harm than good, have attempted to separate mental illness from social problems. Yet, how can we tease out what is social and what is emotional?

Secondly, it is quite evident that most of the breakthroughs in psychopharmacology have happened in the last fifty years of the 1900s. The pace of pharmacological innovations have greatly slowed down and most of the new psychiatric treatments that have come to the market in the last twenty years have been modifications of previous molecules, despite millions of dollars being currently invested into pharmaceutical research.

Thirdly, although we have ample research with functional imaging to identify the exact neurotransmitter and functional changes in specific illnesses, we have been unable to translate this knowledge into clinical practice. For example, we do not have simple tests to measure a person's neurotransmitter levels before prescribing the most appropriate medication. Prescribing thus still follows a trial-and-error method, based on an algorithm formed by consensus guidelines, not truly tailored to an individual's unique biology. Unfortunately, people with treatment-resistant conditions often suffer for years before finding a treatment that can alleviate their suffering.

Finally, as I have mentioned before, our current brain-based model struggles to integrate psychiatry and psychology into a unified whole. With psychiatry basing its treatments in brain sciences and psychology dealing with the mind, we have no way around the paradox of brain-mind dualism as it exists today.

A quantum mental health model addresses all these shortcomings. By acknowledging layers of being and the primacy of consciousness, we can let go of mind-brain dualism and embrace an all-encompassing model of treatment, including a variety of techniques described in this section.

Emerging technologies: Precise diagnosis with QEEG

Fortunately, we are increasingly learning more about consciousness and the brain. The brain, like all matter, is quantum in nature and expresses its actions in the form of both waves and particles, on many different levels. The electroencephalogram or EEG is a trace of the brain's activity. It was invented in the 1940s by psychiatrist Hans Berger, but it was quickly discarded by psychiatrists a couple of decades later as being of no value, perhaps spurred by the success of the neurochemical hypotheses and the promise of new medicines.

It is undeniable that the brain is quantum in nature, as it operates on many different levels. On one level, molecules called neurotransmitters affect our emotion and thinking. On another level, the brain expresses itself through electrical activity, or brain waves. The amount of different brain waves produced in different brain regions gives us information about how various parts of the brain communicate amongst each other and integrate as a whole. In technical parlance, this is called the connectivity of the brain networks.

New algorithms have made it possible to interpret brain waves in terms of amount and connectivity, then compare it to a database of "normal" brains to determine how the particular brain's functioning can be improved. This technique, called Quantitative EEG or Brain mapping, is gradually gathering more and more evidence to not only predict the most effective medication a person is likely to respond to, but also to predict the appropriate training protocols to improve brain connectivity. In this way, different brain regions are able to "talk to" each other and function as an integrated whole.

The emerging field of Pharmaco-EEG (medication prediction on the basis of QEEG), along with the field of pharmacogenomics (predicting the metabolism of medications by the body), has led to the dawn of Precision Psychiatry. Although currently a small movement, as more and more evidence accumulates, every individual will be able to receive truly personalised treatment based on his/her own biology, and not merely based on consensus guidelines.

Neuroplasticity: Your elastic brain

Until recently, we believed that adult neurons were unable to regenerate themselves and that any loss of function of the brain was irreversible. Research over the last two decades has challenged this assumption. Norman Doidge, Canadian psychiatrist, has popularised the concept of neuroplasticity. In his books, *The Brain's Way of Healing* and *The Brain that Changes Itself*, he describes cutting-edge research that exploits the brain's ability to regenerate or compensate for any loss of function.

The fact is that neuroplasticity is at play throughout our lives. What we do or experience repeatedly literally gets wired into our brains. Mental illnesses are the result of neuroplastic changes brought about by genetics, early childhood, life experiences, stress, social factors, and a myriad of other factors all around us. The good news is that the same neuroplasticity can be harnessed to treat these conditions by driving the brain back to its normal operation through neuroplastic change.

Canadian psychologist Donald Hebb proposed that "Neurons that fire together, wire together", meaning that activities that occur together strengthen their connection over time. Michael Merzenich, a prominent researcher of neuroplasticity, believes that the concept of a single drug being the solution for conditions as complex as schizophrenia or depression is simplistic to say the least. In his book *Soft Wired: How the new science of brain plasticity can change your life,* he states that "there is a far greater prospect for achieving neurological recovery through brain training designed to reverse many distorting changes that are part of the illness."

Neurostimulation and Neuromodulation

Increasingly, the field of psychiatry is incorporating the concept of neurostimulation and neuromodulation to effectively manage psychiatric conditions. Neurostimulation is a form of treatment where we directly stimulate the brain or a specific nerve through electric or magnetic fields. Neuromodulation, on the other hand, is a non-invasive form of tweaking brainwaves in specific brain regions to improve various brain functions and connectivity.

I. Electroconvulsive therapy:

One of the earliest and still most effective forms of neurostimulation is electroconvulsive therapy, or ECT, which involves passing a miniscule amount of current through the brain, effectively boosting neurotransmitters and in effect "rebooting" the brain. ECT, unlike what popular myths suggest, does not "fry the brain" but rather has been shown to have a neuroprotective effect. This method boosts the production of BDNF, which is a potent nerve-growth factor. However, due to the risks of memory problems and risks of anaesthesia, ECT is reserved for the most severe spectrum of mental illnesses. People who experience significant somatic symptoms like loss of energy, loss of weight, early morning awakening, and, in particular, melancholic or psychotic symptoms are usually likely to have a good response to ECT, while those with comorbid personality disorders or psychosocial problems are less likely to respond positively.

A client of mine, Mike, was a fifty-eight-year-old farmer in rural New South Wales. He had previously had an episode of depression in his thirties which improved with antidepressants alone. However, he became progressively depressed without any apparent stress to the point that he was complaining of fatigue, lack of motivation, lack of appetite, and hopelessness about the future. He started expressing beliefs that he was contaminated by a chemical he had used on his farm and that he and his family were going to die as a result. He failed to respond to two trials of antidepressants and finally consented to a course of ECT. He experienced marked improvement in his mood, energy levels, and sleep by the end of the course and no longer held the beliefs that he was contaminated.

II. Transcranial magnetic stimulation:

More recently, transcranial magnetic stimulation, or TMS, is gaining popularity as an effective treatment for depression and some anxiety disorders, like obsessive compulsive disorder and post-traumatic stress disorder. TMS involves applying a magnetic field on the brain cortex, which produces localised electrical activity in the cortex but does not cause seizures or loss of consciousness, unlike ECT. Not requiring anaesthesia, it can be performed in an outpatient setting and is thus a highly appealing form of treatment.

On the downside, treatments have to be administered daily for several weeks until remission, to be followed by maintenance treatment for relapse prevention. It is suggested as a treatment when two antidepressants have been ineffective, however, it is less effective than a course of ECT.

My client, David was a forty-five-year-old executive who had developed depression and anxiety in the context of workplace stress. He tried several antidepressants but was exquisitely sensitive to their side effects, thus he could not even reach therapeutic doses of medications. He had tried psychotherapy for several years but there was not much improvement in his symptoms. We decided to try TMS, given its safety profile and lack of side effects. David experienced significant improvement in his depression and anxiety within a month of treatment.

Despite the common view that ECT and TMS are the only neurostimulatory or neuromodulatory techniques available in psychiatry, there are in fact a variety of other well-researched but little-known techniques that are increasingly finding their way into your friendly psychiatrist or psychologist's office.

III. Transcranial direct current stimulation (tDCS)

This involves passing miniscule amounts of current through the scalp while a patient is conscious. Unlike ECT, which uses current in the range of milliamperes, the current passed in tDCS is in the range of microamperes, such as that produced by a nine-volt battery. Thus it does not produce seizures or loss of consciousness, and the person undergoing treatment experiences only mild tingling sensations around the electrode. tDCS works by reducing the resting membrane potential of the brain in the cortex below the area of stimulation. In a sense, it makes the brain more responsive to stimuli. While in itself it is not a powerful form of treatment, it can be a powerful adjuvant when combined with other neuromodulatory techniques. This can be compared to the melting of plastic to make it more pliable, after which the brain is easier to shape through other techniques, whether psychotherapy, neurofeedback or TMS.

Because of its simplicity, non-invasiveness and lack of side effects, tDCS has been investigated in fields as diverse as anxiety, PTSD, depression, pain, and even to enhance creativity. Snyder and Chi found that most subjects they recruited in their 2012 study were unable to solve the famous nine-dot problem initially. The nine-dot problem is a puzzle, wherein you are asked to join all the dots with four straight lines without taking the pen off the page. It requires out-of-the-box thinking to solve. When the investigators applied tDCS to the right anterior temporal lobe, more than 40% of participants could solve the problem! Of course, this does not imply that anyone can zap themselves with a nine-volt battery and see results, but administration of tDCS by trained personnel can augment conventional treatment methods.

A special mention about the role of tDCS in managing chronic pain: chronic pain is a classic example of the brain's plasticity gone rogue. The pain threshold is reset so that even stimuli that were previously innocuous produce incredible pain. tDCS enables one to reactivate and re-modulate the brain's plasticity—thus, it potentially resets the pain threshold and has been found to be extremely effective in migraines and a variety of chronic pain conditions, especially neuropathic or nerve pain.

I was first introduced to tDCS a few years back in a workshop. The device is so small that it can fit in the palm of your hand. I got my friend, who suffered from tinnitus, to try a few sessions. Initially, he did not notice anything except for a strange tingling and itchiness on the left side of his forehead, where the cathode was placed. The sensation subsided soon. After a few sessions, he reported marked improvement in his tinnitus.

IV. Cranial Electro Stimulation (CES):

Cranial electrostimulation involves delivering a small, pulsed, alternating current via electrodes on the head, mastoid process, or earlobes. It was invented in the Soviet Union in the 1950s and spread rapidly through Europe, Japan, and the United States. To date there have been hundreds of studies on the use of CES for anxiety, depression, insomnia, and pain, demonstrating significant benefits. It is widely used in the U.S. army for PTSD. CES is proposed to stimulate brain regions associated with key neurotransmitters and has been shown to increase serotonin and beta endorphins in the central nervous system. Quantitative EEG reports show it decreases delta waves while increasing alpha waves, fostering a sense of calm and well-being. Being quite effective for anxiety and insomnia, it often enables people who rely heavily on benzodiazepines and other sleep medications to reduce such use. They have also been found to be helpful to reduce craving in substance use, especially alcohol use. Long-term daily use for a few weeks can be quite effective in improving sleep and anxiety, according to several randomised controlled trials.

I was fortunate enough to try CES with Dave Siever, the founder of Mind Alive, a company that designs and manufactures equipment for improving brain performance. The device—again, like tDCS—is so small that it fits into the palm of your hand. Dave rubbed some saline onto my earlobes to attach the electrodes, and he urged me to sit down for the session, as it can sometimes cause dizziness and vertigo. I felt calm and my mood picked up after a few minutes, like a high after a good workout. Now I knew why it was so effective for reducing substance use—this was like a natural high on the body's own chemicals! I did feel a bit dizzy, as I had put the machine on the longest pulse, but there were no major side effects. Given its effectiveness—at least in mild cases—and lack of side effects, CES is here to stay.

IV. Transcutaneous vagus nerve stimulation (tVNS):

The vagus nerve is the most intriguing cranial nerve of the body. It is the longest cranial nerve which traverses the whole body, and is thus called the wanderer of the body. The vagus nerve forms what is commonly referred to as the gut-brain axis, a signalling system between the gastrointestinal tract and the central nervous system, which forms the basis of a large part of our body's immune system. It has long been the focus of psychoneuroimmunology, a branch of medicine focusing on the complex interrelationships between the mind, nervous system, endocrine system, and the immune system. Since the 1960s, the vagus has also been recognised as an important mediator of the relaxation response and plays a key role in emotional regulation as well.

Vagus nerve stimulation has been used for decades to manage epilepsy and also sometimes refractory depression. In conventional vagus nerve stimulation, a stimulator needs to be surgically implanted close to the vagus nerve at the neck. The invasiveness of this procedure has so far precluded it from becoming mainstream and is restricted to treat only the most severely ill and refractory cases.

More recently, transcutaneous vagus nerve stimulation, or tVNS, has been found to be just as effective in managing some conditions like depression and migraines. The vagus nerve can either be stimulated at the neck or through an earlobe, which contains the auricular branch of the vagus nerve (the most accessible part of the nerve). Although still in the research phase, tVNS seems to be a promising new treatment for conditions not usually responsive to medications, like fibromyalgia and autoimmune disorders, due to the vagus's role in immune mediation. Preliminary studies also suggest that it might help in developmental trauma disorder or complex post-traumatic stress disorder.

There are a lot of tVNS devices on the market, and many have been approved for migraine and tinnitus treatment. My preliminary research was with a device called Nervana, which is classified as a wellness device. It stimulates the auditory division of the vagus nerve in the ear canal through a pair of headphones, which you can do while listening to music. A thirty-minute session left me feeling calm, as if I had just meditated during that time. I sometimes use the Nervana if I am feeling stressed out and am not in a meditation-friendly environment. Although this is not a medical-grade device—and I am far from recommending it for managing mental health issues—I intend to illustrate with this example the ease with which tVNS can soon become a part of mental health interventions.

V. Auditory Neuromodulation

Since ancient times, the concept of healing through sound has been a part of many cultures. Hindus have been chanting mantras and Tibetans have been chanting and using singing bowls and prayer wheels for centuries to achieve better health and higher states of consciousness.

Research on brain waves shows that a particular repetitive sound frequency can cause brainwaves to resonate at the same frequency, a concept called brainwave entrainment. Further, we also know that when two different sound frequencies are presented to the two ears, the brain actually hears a single sound—at a frequency which is the difference between the two original frequencies—and entrains to this new frequency. These sound waves, or binaural beats, are now a part of popular culture, and YouTube is abound in music with binaural beats incorporated. Binaural beats are intended to produce specific wave patterns—alpha for relaxed awareness, beta for alertness and concentration, theta for deeper states and meditation, or even gamma, to encourage higher states of consciousness. While there has been some research into the use of binaural beats, its area of application has been mainly in enhancing peak performance or inducing relaxation rather than specific mental health conditions.

Auditory neuromodulation is a very diverse field and the reader should by no means assume that it is limited to binaural beats. Here I will describe some of the applications which have been backed by a significant body of research.

Integrated Listening System and Tomatis Method:

In the early 1950s, Dr Alfred Tomatis, an ear, nose, and throat physician, invented the Electronic ear, which re-educated and restored the singer's deficient voice qualities. Gradually, Tomatis expanded his research to treat developmental conditions like learning and communication disorders, delays in speech and language development, autism, ADHD, and sensory integration issues as well as depression and stress. He realised that training the right ear to discriminate and detect sound changes could ultimately help improve overall personal growth and social interaction. The Tomatis method has several phases, with the first phase beginning with listening to filtered music for an hour or two hours every day for ten to fifteen days, followed by further phases tailored to the individual. The Tomatis method is now available in seventy-five countries, has around 2000 practitioners around the world, and is shown to have beneficial effects in some developmental conditions in case reports and small studies.

Another sound therapy based on similar principles is the **Integrated Listening Systems** program, developed in 2007 by sound therapists Ron Minson, Kate O'Brien Minson, and Randall Redfield. It has been claimed to reduce sensitivity to sound and improve a child's ability to process sound and control emotions, thus improving behaviour, social skills, and concentration. It has been used for developmental conditions like autism, ADHD, and sensory processing disorders.

The Integrated Listening Systems program involves a child listening to classical music that has been modified to emphasise particular frequencies. The child uses special headphones that can conduct sound through bone as well as through air. At the same time as listening to the music, the child does balance, coordination, and visual exercises. The program involves thirty- to sixty-minute sessions two to five times a week for up to six months. Although backed by anecdotal evidence, there is lack of quality research to say confidently whether it is effective in these developmental conditions.

Safe and Sound Protocol

The vagus nerve, which I talked about in a previous section, has a role in our psychological defence as well. Dr. Stephen Porges, professor of psychiatry at the University of North Carolina, shed light on the role of the vagus in our emotional life when he proposed the Polyvagal theory in 1994. According to the theory, the vagus nerve includes three distinct circuits that define the ways in which organisms can respond to their environment. The vagal circuits activate in a hierarchical fashion—from the developmentally newest to oldest. In addition, each circuit can override the others. The newest circuit, a branch of the ventral vagus, promotes social interactions through a calming effect and the stimulation of speech and the facial muscles. The next older circuit, another branch of the ventral vagus, mediates the traditional fight-or-flight response of the sympathetic nervous system. The oldest circuit, the dorsal vagus, activates in extremely dangerous situations and can cause a person to freeze.

Clinically, the polyvagal theory helps us understand many psychiatric illnesses. The newest part of the vagus is called the social engagement system. This allows you to enjoy social interactions and connect with people. The second part kicks in when there is perceived danger and initiates the classic flight or fight response. Gone awry, our nervous systems perceive threats even when there are none and results in an anxiety response which, when chronic, leads to anxiety disorders.

The dorsal vagus or the primitive part allows an organism to "play dead" when there is inescapable danger. Children who suffer severe abuse in their childhood, especially at the hands of their caregivers, probably engage the dorsal vagus which helps them shut down physically or dissociate from the traumatic experience. This is the brain region that is constantly engaged in people who develop post-traumatic stress disorder. This is also a key brain area in autism, where sensory overload results in a shut down.

Based on four decades of research on the polyvagal theory, Stephen Porges has developed the Safe and Sound Protocol, which is a five-day auditory intervention designed to reduce stress and auditory sensitivity while enhancing social engagement and resilience. The SSP uses the auditory system as a portal to the vagus nerve complex. It involves listening to specially processed music for an hour a day for five consecutive days. The music trains the auditory pathways by focusing on the frequency envelope of human speech. It is claimed to improve the overall functioning of the vagus nerve to improve self-soothing and autonomic regulation. There is considerable research on the use of SSP to improve functioning in conditions like autism, sensory processing disorders, post-traumatic stress disorders, and anxiety disorders. It is not a stand-alone therapy, but forms a platform to improve the effectiveness of other neuroplastic interventions.

Alice was a thirty- year-old woman who had suffered terrible abuse during her childhood. She was hypervigilant, got startled at any little noise, and reported high levels of anxiety throughout the day. Her sleep was interrupted by nightmares of her past and she was exhausted during the day. She had tried a variety of therapies without much success. She underwent the five-day SSP therapy. On day four, she reported feeling calmer and said she slept better at night. By the fifth day, Alice was less anxious and more engaged, ready to move on to the next stage of treatment.

BAUD and RESET therapy:

The Bio-acoustical utilization device (BAUD) is a simple device which generates a droning sound, much like a hive of bees. This little device, invented by Dr. Frank Lawlis, has been used with success in a variety of conditions, especially anxiety, PTSD, and eating disorders. Dr. George Lindenfeld, a clinical psychologist who has spent years working with war veterans in the United States, developed the RESET therapy (Reconsolidation and Enhancement through Stimulation of Emotional Triggers) to specifically treat people with PTSD. In RESET therapy, the BAUD is used to disrupt the neural pathways in the amygdala through sound. These neural pathways maintain the symptoms of PTSD, like nightmares and flashbacks.

The results are, frankly, quite impressive. Dr. Lindenfeld has published case reports and case series of veterans with PTSD who have shown marked improvement in symptoms after just four sessions of RESET therapy, to the point that some of them no longer met criteria for PTSD. His research is backed by pre- and post-therapy QEEG showing normalisation of the brain regions involved in PTSD symptoms.

I am fortunate enough to have had some training in RESET therapy under Dr. Lindenfeld. The results in my clinical practice have been quite dramatic. Clients who presented with ongoing symptoms of PTSD reported diminution of their symptoms after just one or two sessions. I am yet to come across any therapy or medication that reduces symptoms so rapidly. In addition, the improvements were sustained over time. I believe that Dr. Lindenfeld is definitely on to something. More recently, he has expanded his arena to use RESET therapy in complex PTSD, or developmental trauma disorder, with positive results.

Allison was a sixteen-year-old girl who came to see me at the insistence of her mother. She had been molested a year ago and now had persistent flashbacks and nightmares of the incident. She was also getting frequent panic attacks and had started avoiding school. When she came to see me she was very anxious, as previously she had been asked in therapy to discuss the abuse, a standard part of current assessment in therapy. When I told her that she need not share her trauma with me and the therapy we would be doing was non-verbal, she heaved a sigh of relief. As she put the headphones on, I asked her to focus on the memory while I turned the knobs on the device to disrupt the fear circuitry. We continued this for twenty minutes, following which I asked her to try to evoke the memory again. "I can't see it!" she said, quite relieved. On follow-up, she described that the nightmares had reduced and she was having fewer panic attacks. Her mother reported that Allison seemed calmer and happier in school.

Audio-visual entrainment (AVE)

Audio-visual entrainment, as the name implies, uses flashing lights and pulsing tones to gently guide the brain into specific brain wave patterns, like deep meditation, relaxation, and even concentration. When the brain is exposed to rhythmic tones, brain waves get "entrained", that is they resonate to the same frequency generated by the tone. The combination with visual stimulation makes the entrainment more powerful. It also increases cerebral blood flow and increases glucose metabolism. AVE was first discovered by Adrian and Matthews in 1934 and since then has developed into a sophisticated science. Thus you can entrain your brain waves to be in the state that you want to be in. For those with fatigue or poor concentration, AVE in the beta frequency will increase energy, while for those suffering from poor sleep, AVE in the alpha or theta will induce deep relaxation and sleep. AVE has been used to treat a variety of conditions including Attention deficit disorder, anxiety, PTSD, chronic pain, and fibromyalgia. It has also been used for peak-performance training.

Although there are several AVE devices on the market, The DAVID Delight by Mind Alive is backed by good research. Their website cites over twenty studies which have been done in a variety of conditions using the DAVID (digital audio visual integration) devices.

DAVID Delight is an easy-to-use AVE device. As it uses both auditory and visual stimulation, it requires the use of headphones and a special set of glasses that pass flashing lights through the eyes in sync with the auditory frequencies. It has a few different preset programs, like meditation, relaxation, and concentration. I have used it to improve my concentration and boost creativity. During the first five minutes of my first session, I was getting a few creative solutions to a problem I had been working on for a while! The one caution I would recommend is for people with light sensitivities, especially epilepsy, to be wary of the flashing lights. Otherwise, it is very safe and easy to use.

VI. Photobiomodulation

We have long known that light can influence our mood, and light therapy is used to treat seasonal affective disorders. This light is usually in the visible spectrum and goes in through the eyes to produce the desired effect. Recent research shows that light need not be presented through our eyes to produce an effect. Light is, in fact, absorbed through our skin and can be used to treat a variety of conditions. This emerging field is called photobiomodulation—modulating our chemistry through light. Infrared or near-infrared light of different wavelengths has been used for quicker post-surgical healing, improving blood flow, and in improving brain functioning.

Contrary to popular belief, our skulls are actually permeable to this wavelength of light. In addition, researchers have found that light applied through the nasal passage directly reaches the base of the brain, a site which is difficult to access through other non-invasive neurostimulation techniques. It is thus a promising technique for conditions related to deep brain pathology.

One of the primary players in brain photobiomodulation is Vielight, a Canadian organisation which developed transcranial and intranasal devices that deliver pulsed, 810 nanometres, near-infrared light in 2011. The Neuro Gamma delivers pulsed light at 40 Hz and is believed to entrain brainwaves to this frequency. An article by Zomorrodi et al. in Nature, a leading academic journal, reports that a single session of twenty minutes using the Neuro Gamma increased high-frequency brain waves of alpha, beta, and gamma while decreasing low frequencies. This explains the positive effect it has on cognition and improving functioning in brain injury and degenerative conditions. The Neuro Alpha is a similar device which delivers the pulsed light at 10 Hz, designed to improve overall brain metabolism and produce a state of calm awareness. It is a promising new approach, given the lack of side effects and the ease of use; all one has to do is put the helmet on, clip the nasal prong in one of the nasal passages, and turn the unit on. It is designed to turn off automatically after twenty minutes, eliminating the risk of inadvertent overuse.

There have been robust clinical reports on the potential of the Vielight Neuro Gamma to modify the pathology of Alzheimer's disease. In June 2019, Vielight started a large multi-site clinical trial across Canada and the U.S. investigating the effect of the Neuro Gamma on subjects with moderate to severe cognitive impairment due to Alzheimer's disease. This trial is expected to run till 2021. It is indeed a promising technology, so watch for the results of this study.

My experience with the Vielight Neuro Gamma is so far limited, but I came across a mental health professional who had himself used the Neuro Gamma for a month for a declining memory and reported considerable relief in symptoms. Other professionals use it everyday during meditation to achieve elevated states of consciousness, which occur when more gamma brainwaves are being produced. One of my clients with early cognitive decline described considerable improvement in his memory with regular use for a month.

VII. Pulsed Electromagnetic Field (PEMF)

PEMF is a technology which uses continuous trains of low-voltage alternating currents within coils, which create a weak electromagnetic field over the treatment area. PEMF has been used for many years now in the field of injury management. It has been shown to increase the microcirculation of an area and helps in formation of new vessels. PEMF stimulates repair and regeneration of tissues and has been used in conditions like fractures and osteoarthritis. However, recent research indicates that it can also be useful in mental health conditions like depression and anxiety. A study conducted at Harvard Medical School in 2014 found that there was a greater than 10% improvement in mood after a single, twenty-minute PEMF session in patients with major depression and bipolar disorder. Another study found 62% reduction in depression rating after five weeks of PEMF treatment, and in another study, there was a 73% remission rate after eight weeks of treatment. These results are comparable to responses to standard antidepressant treatment. Although we do need more research to replicate these findings, it seems to be a promising treatment, especially as it can be easily adapted to home use and is not known to cause any significant side effects. Moreover, it improves the quality of sleep, which is usually more difficult to treat with antidepressants alone.

In the next chapters, we will explore the mental and emotional bodies and a range of healing modalities for them.

Chapter 11

THE MENTAL BODY

"The world as we have created it is a process of our thinking. It cannot be changed without changing our thinking."

—Albert Einstein

The next levels that most people are familiar with are the emotional and mental bodies. Conventionally both are referred to as the mind, but I like to distinguish between the two as there are different approaches to heal these different aspects. Emotions and thoughts are linked to each other like the proverbial chicken and egg. Some theorists believe that thoughts generate emotions, while more recent research suggests that actually emotions are generated first and thoughts are attached to it later.

Psychotherapy addresses both the emotional and mental bodies. However, for the sake of clarity, I will first discuss some techniques that focus on the mental body and then move on to the emotional body. The reader might notice that I am actually working backwards, beginning with the mental body, and then the emotional and vital layers. This is because mental techniques are better known, and a lot of people might be already familiar with them. It will be easier to tackle these first, then discuss some of the lesser-known techniques used to treat the emotional and vital layers.

I. Psychoanalysis and Psychodynamic psychotherapy:

The oldest form of psychotherapy since the time of Freud, these therapies need little elaboration. The terms are often used interchangeably, but psychodynamic therapy is a briefer version. They are based on the theory that the subconscious houses a lot of our repressed memories and impulses, which unconsciously determine our day-to-day behaviour. The aim of therapy is to become more aware of our unconscious motivations and impulses and understand how our past influences our present, especially in terms of recreating relationship patterns. For example, a person who was abused by his father as a child might see all older males as punitive and this might affect their current interpersonal relationships. These therapies, along with a variety of adaptations, are based on the concept of free association (the person is encouraged to say what comes to his mind uncensored), and the therapist provides interpretations to help a person access their unconscious motivations. Such therapy is quite intensive, often requiring weekly or twice-weekly therapy for several years before people are able to progress. Often, fragile people find it quite challenging to process the memories and emotions dredged up in the process and tend to drop out of therapy early. These therapies are more for the psychologically-minded, who are fairly functional and want to seek a greater understanding of themselves and their motivations.

II. Cognitive Therapy:

Championed by Aaron Beck, an American psychiatrist, cognitive therapy rapidly gained popularity in the 1980s onwards. The basis for cognitive therapy is the premise that negative automatic thoughts influence our emotions and certain habitual patterns of cognitive thinking can eventually lead to a variety of mental disorders, like anxiety and depression. Cognitive therapy is more goal-directed than psychodynamic therapy, and thus more economical in terms of time. It deals with more "here and now" problems; thus it appeals to a lot of people who want to address just their current issues and not necessarily delve into their childhood. Of course, there is also the option of more intense therapy, delving into the core "schema" that influence our behaviour. Schema are like our internal programming codes which determine our thoughts and behaviours.

Behaviour therapy was originally created by B.F. Skinner, an American psychologist, and other scientists based on laboratory experiments focusing on behavioural conditioning. All animals learn behaviours based on common learning theories. Classical conditioning involves pairing one stimulus with another to increase the likelihood of them occurring together. Operant conditioning, on the other hand, involves rewarding or punishing behaviours to increase or decrease the likelihood of occurrence. Modern therapies combine principles from both schools and are thus called cognitive behaviour therapy (CBT).

All in all, cognitive behaviour therapy is quite a practical and manualised type of therapy which is relatively simple to implement and thus highly flexible and adaptable. Increasingly, time and cost restrictions have led to the development of internet-based CBT programs like Moodgym (an online self-help program), as well as workbook- or module-based programs. There are a lot of programs available, but I particularly like the modules from Centre for Clinical Intervention, an organization based in Western Australia, which has self-learning modules for many disorders along with worksheets and information leaflets. They are all free to the public and extremely well-researched. Another great self-help resource for CBT is David Burns's "Feeling

Good', which is a very user-friendly step by step program of self-help using CBT.

CBT is easily the most widely prevalent therapy today. It has been adapted to address specific issues like eating disorders, alcohol dependence, and other substance use disorders. Although widely successful, there are areas that CBT has only limited benefit in—for example, post-traumatic stress disorder, complex post-traumatic stress disorder, and personality disorders. In some areas, like eating disorders and substance use, it has only modest benefits.

III. Interpersonal therapy:

Obviously our emotions are largely influenced by our relationships, a thought which forms an important focus of psychological treatment. Interpersonal therapy (IPT) is a phased, manualized treatment focusing on a person's relationships and addresses various interpersonal issues which could lead to depression. IPT is very useful when psychological problems are related to role conflicts (for example, between partners), role transitions (for example, postpartum depression), or grief, whether over loss of a loved one, loss of functioning, or loss of some ideal. It is practical and solution-focused, so is usually suitable for someone who was reasonably well-functioning before a particular event or loss caused their depression.

IV. Mindfulness:

Mindfulness draws on the ancient Buddhist and Zen traditions and is a technique to bring our awareness consciously into the present. It is the practice of purposely bringing our attention to our present experience, without judgement. Most of our lives we spend in the past, reliving past events, conversations, regretting things we have done or steps we have failed to take, and beating ourselves up over our bad decisions. While CBT can be an effective tool to challenge these negative beliefs, another solution is to keep our awareness on the present moment and be mindful in everything we do. Mindfulness is an entirely different way of being, rather than doing. There is ample research which shows the benefits of mindfulness on brain neuroplasticity. It literally changes the brain and floods it with feel-good neurotransmitters. There are various offshoots of mindfulness, like mindfulness-based stress reduction and mindfulness based cognitive therapy, which can complement cognitive strategies very effectively.

These well-known therapies are the mainstay of current psychological treatment. However, although effective in a lot of conditions, they tend to fall short when it comes to complex mental health conditions. Thus, it is necessary to be aware of techniques which work on the emotional and vital bodies, which are discussed next.

Chapter 12

THE EMOTIONAL BODY

"No, this trick won't work... How on earth are you going to explain in terms of chemistry and physics so important a biological phenomenon as first love?"

—Albert Einstein

Despite the range of therapies available—which I have mentioned in the previous chapter, and which are very useful for addressing mental disorders—I find that there remains a significant subset of people with complex mental health issues who do not respond well to therapy, despite years of treatment. These are the people who have had significant trauma or neglect in their lives, and this affects every area of their lives. Post-traumatic stress disorder is a well-known condition which one usually associates with combat veterans, first responders, or those who have been in some terrible accident. However, there is also a population who have suffered extensive abuse or neglect, especially in their early years. Noted psychiatrist and trauma expert Bessel van der Kolk proposed the term Developmental Trauma Disorder in 2009. It is characterised by dysregulation of emotions, behaviour, self-concept, and relations, in addition to symptoms of PTSD. The development of the brain is normally from bottom upwards. When stress responses—due to abuse or neglect—are repeated over an extended period in childhood, this sequential development is disrupted and connections between the limbic (emotional) brain and higher brain centres are not well-formed. These are people, among many others, who will need help integrating their emotional and mental bodies. One of the ways to do this is through limbic therapy.

I. Limbic therapy:

Trauma memories are intimately lodged in the limbic system or emotional brain, which is the earliest part of the brain to develop. It is thus difficult to access this part of the brain through words, which are processed through the neocortex or executive centre of the brain. This explains why PTSD cannot be treated through cognitive strategies alone. A woman who was injured in a car accident says, "I have gone through months of therapy and challenged all my negative cognitions, but every time I get into the driver's seat, I get a panic attack." If the trauma happened in childhood, when the brain was still growing, the limbic system essentially goes rogue and is not under control of the higher cortical centres.

Bessel van der Kolk has coined the term "limbic therapy" for those therapies which directly access the limbic system and address the emotional dysregulation and traumatic memories. In his book, *The Body Keeps The Score,* he outlines how trauma memories are trapped in the body and thus respond better to body-oriented therapies. I believe that these memories are trapped in the emotional body, which is why they are released through therapies like neurofeedback, EMDR, and yoga, among others. Some of the limbic therapies are explained below:

Neurofeedback:

Neurofeedback is one such neuromodulatory technique which accesses the limbic system. Also called neurotherapy or EEG biofeedback, it is a type of biofeedback that uses sensors on the scalp to measure brain waves and displays it on a computer screen to provide direct feedback to the brain about its functioning. Neurofeedback is based on the principle of operant conditioning: rewarding optimal brain wave frequencies while inhibiting undesirable frequencies, through the use of visual and auditory rewards. The brain is thus encouraged to produce more appropriate brain activity for better self-regulation. With regular sessions, the brain learns to be in a more efficient physiological state and forms new connections; thus, different parts of the brain start communicating better. I like to describe neurofeedback as gym training for the brain—and as with gym training, it can take twenty, forty, or even more sessions to produce significant improvement. Yet, for people who have gone through years and years of talk therapy without success, the results can be quite dramatic. Trauma expert Bessel van der Kolk demonstrated a 40% increase in executive function in formerly "untreatable" adults with histories of developmental trauma after twenty-four sessions of neurofeedback.

My journey into neurofeedback began in 2017 when, frustrated with the limitations of conventional therapy, I came across van der Kolk's book. Synchronously enough, I was able to attend a workshop on neurofeedback at the Service for Rehabilitation and Treatment of Torture and Trauma survivors (STARTTS) in early 2018. There I met Mirjana Askovic, a reputed neurotherapist who works with refugees with PTSD in Sydney. Askovic inspired me to train in neurofeedback myself.

Nothing convinces one more than a positive personal experience. As part of my training, I had to do several sessions of self-regulation. During those days, I was burning both ends of the candle and perpetually exhausted. I was surviving on 4 cups of coffee a day and felt like my brain was always sleeping. On the first day of training, I used a stimulating protocol to gently nudge my brain to awaken. After a few minutes, I felt like a fog had lifted from my mind! Everything around me seemed brighter and more alive. It was like going back to my teens, when I was full of energy! That evening I was extremely productive, yet able to relax and fall asleep naturally! Having tried every available trick of the trade (from health supplements to antidepressants) unsuccessfully, I knew that this was a therapy that worked. I still continue to use neurofeedback to improve my cognition.

Clients with a history of trauma are naturally reluctant to rehash their traumatic memories repeatedly in therapy, and are usually relieved to know that they need not discuss their trauma during neurofeedback sessions. Yet, trauma processing occurs quite naturally during the sessions, as the brain becomes "unstuck". Clients I treat with neurofeedback describe how calm they feel during and after sessions and how well they sleep after sessions. Unlike conventional therapies (which they often dread, as they liken it to opening Pandora's box), they tell me that they look forward to neurofeedback sessions. Here, they are able to experience relaxation, often for the first time in their lives.

There are several varieties of neurofeedback, with the most common and most research-backed being amplitude neurofeedback. Another promising type is infra-low neurofeedback, which trains subcortical potentials generated by astrocytes (which regulate rhythms related to mood, energy, and concentration). Infra-low neurofeedback is particularly effective for improving network connectivity between various brain regions, which are often disrupted in long-standing conditions like ADHD, autism spectrum, complex PTSD, and attachment issues.

There is increasing research into neurofeedback not only to treat conditions like PTSD and ADHD, but also chronic conditions like autism, traumatic brain injury, and schizophrenia. In fact, neurofeedback is also being used in peak-performance training by elite athletes, Olympic teams, and corporate leaders who want to learn to be in a state of flow: completely immersed, energised and enjoying the present moment We are indeed in an exciting new era as advances in technology allow more quantitative research into the applications of neurofeedback.

Eye Movement Desensitisation and Reprocessing (EMDR):

EMDR is another limbic therapy which has gathered a substantial body of evidence especially regarding efficacy in PTSD and developmental trauma. The name might sound formidable, but the therapy itself is neither formidable nor complicated. The client is asked to recall a specific trauma and the therapist asks her to follow his fingers with her eyes. The therapist then directs the movements of the client's eyes from side to side. These eye movements are hypothesised to reprocess the memory in such a way that it loses its emotional valence. The process might need to be repeated several times according to the degree of emotional distress it causes. A new positive cognition is integrated into the client's psyche using similar finger movements. EMDR has long been mired in controversy, mostly because it almost seems magical that wiggling a finger in front of a person's eyes can help process trauma. There is now considerable, high-quality evidence to prove that it is not inferior to CBT in treatment of trauma. However, superiority over CBT has been harder to prove, as deterrents are quick to point out the shortcomings of studies conducted.

EMDR has always intrigued me, so I attended a training with a prominent EMDR therapist. The big name and the finger wiggling had always daunted me, so it was a relief to discover that it was actually a therapy which was easy to apply to clinical practice. To get an experience of sessions, we worked in pairs to work on our own minor traumas. It was quite a revelation to me how it helped me focus on bodily sensations and helped release not just the sensations but the associated negative memories.

Recently, some practitioners have started combining limbic therapies, especially neurofeedback and EMDR, to achieve optimal results for clients. While some choose to start with neurofeedback to regulate the brain before moving on to EMDR, others use them in a more laissez faire manner.

Brain Spotting:

Brain Spotting is a relatively new therapy developed in 2003 by David Grand, a social worker, to address symptoms of PTSD. According to Grand, the direction in which people look or gaze can affect the way they feel. The therapist guides the eyes of the client to find appropriate "brainspots", or an eye position that activates a traumatic memory or painful emotion. Both EMDR and brain spotting use visual fields to process stored memory and rewire the brain. Brainspotting is considered to be more flexible and the therapist follows the client's natural direction, without needing to stick to a protocol. Practitioners mention that brain spotting tends to work at a faster rate than EMDR, but being an emerging therapy, research so far is still limited, although promising.

II. Heart Coherence:

We have intuitively known for centuries that the heart is the seat of feelings. Even to this day, we use heart symbols to depict love and use terms like "heartfelt" or "from the bottom of my heart" to describe our true emotions. Yet, since the 19th century, the heart was merely regarded as a powerful pump whose only job was to circulate blood to all parts of the body and make sure it was well-oxygenated. This mechanistic model is still conventionally taught in medical schools. However, we now know many more interesting facts about the heart and the role it plays in our emotional lives. The heart generates the largest electrical field of the body, ten times more powerful than the brain. Not only that—in the last decade, scientists have discovered that the heart actually contains a mini-brain consisting of 40,000 neurons that can send messages to the brain about how the body feels. This heart-brain communicates directly with the limbic system and can modify its state. When a person is relaxed and open, the heart rate varies in a regular pattern, called a coherent state. It appears on a graph as a steady, sine-wave-like pattern. This state of coherence is associated with mental clarity, intuitive ability, and good judgement.

The HeartMath Institute, founded in 1991 by Doc Childre, has been a leader in research into heart coherence and its impact on not only mental health, but also improving creativity, resilience, and spiritual connections. Through a process called the Quick Coherence Technique, we can bring our heart rate variability into a coherent pattern within a matter of a few minutes. The Institute markets small biofeedback devices which help give feedback about a person's heart rate variability and help them move into a state of coherence.

There is an impressive body of evidence on the use of heart rate variability training, or coherence training, on a variety of clinical conditions, including anxiety, depression, PTSD, chronic fatigue, and chronic pain. What I find more impressive, is the extensive research that has been done in schools on children with behavioural problems and ADHD to improve their emotional regulation and impulse control. Many schools in the U.S. have adopted the HeartMath Program for their students with improvement not only in academic performance and exam results, but also in reducing behavioural disturbances.

There are several simple devices available to help improve heart coherence. The Inner Balance is a personal device which can work with your phone or tablet, while professionals can choose to opt for the emWave, which has many additional features to use for multiple clients. I find the emWave extremely useful to teach clients the concept of heart coherence, and get them to practice the Quick Coherence Technique while watching their coherence levels change on the screen. I have had highly agitated clients calm down significantly after ten to twenty minutes of coherence training. Because of its simplicity, it can be used as an adjunct to almost any kind of therapy, and even as a stand-alone practice for high-performing people who want to reduce their overall stress levels.

In the next chapter, we will have a look at techniques which work on the vital or energy body.

Chapter 13

THE ENERGY BODY

"Everything is energy and that's all there is to it. Match the frequency of the reality you want and you cannot help but get that reality. It can be no other way. This is not philosophy. This is physics."

—Albert Einstein

Once in the realm of "alternative medicine", which seemed to be an euphemism for quackery, energy medicine is gaining more recognition in mainstream medicine as we shed our mechanistic concepts of the human body and understand more about the human energy field. Quantum physics explains how we are both energy and matter, although this concept has been slow to permeate into the medical community. Renowned energy medicine researcher James Oschman says that all medicine is energy medicine, as we endeavour to understand how the body produces different energies and how we can apply these energies to benefit the body. Human electric fields have been known and studied for decades, mainly in the heart (what we call the ECG is a measure of the electrical field of the heart) and the brain (the EEG, as discussed earlier, which is the field of brainwaves). More recently, the use of magnetometers has made it possible for us to measure the biomagnetic field, which provides much more information about the functioning of the human body.

In the 1980s, Dr. John Zimmermann of the University of Colorado School of Medicine demonstrated that practitioners of various hands-on and hands-off therapies such as Reiki, Pranic Healing, healing touch, reconnective healing, aura balancing, etc., can emit extremely low-frequency (ELF) electromagnetic signals from their hands, which are not seen in non-practitioners. These frequencies sweep up and down through the range that researchers have found to be effective in stimulating tissue repair. The practitioner's field can induce current flows in individuals in close proximity.

The University of Arizona has used an extra low-frequency meter to measure the flow of energy from Reiki practitioners. The emitted energy was more marked in people at a master level. Researcher Melinda Connor stated that these practitioners were emitting a range of frequencies from 20 Hz to 1000 Hz.

Energy Medicine has a special role in mental illnesses, as these therapies have an interesting role in releasing long-suppressed "somatic" (or "body") memories of trauma and abuse. Noted psychiatrist and trauma researcher Bessel van der Kolk calls developmental trauma the silent epidemic, it is so ubiquitous in our culture today. Trauma that is sustained in childhood is etched into the limbic system as well as the body in the form of somatic memories, which talk-therapies fail to address and energy therapies can help.

The following are some of the energy therapies that have been practiced for some time and have gathered a small body of research evidence. However, it is useful to remember that current medical funding is extremely skewed towards biological therapies and thus, there is scant research into energy therapies in general. The few that are done are often ignored by mainstream medicine.

I. Energy Psychology:

Energy Psychology is an emerging field which focuses on the relationship of thoughts, emotions, and behaviours to the body's bioenergy systems, such as the biofield, chakras, and meridians. Within the discipline of energy psychology exists several therapies, some of which have an impressive evidence base for the treatment of developmental trauma, PTSD, anxiety, and depression. These therapies are sometimes referred to as "power therapies" because they work so quickly compared to traditional talk therapies.

Applied Kinesiology: This was developed by Dr. Goodheart and uses the testing of muscle strength as a diagnostic procedure to indicate the health of bodily functions. It uses the body's subtle energy to reveal any correlation between weakness in certain muscle groups and diseases. Acupuncture points are treated with pressure to alleviate ailments.

Thought Field Therapy: TFT was developed by Dr. Roger Callahan in the 1980s. He developed simple algorithms of tapping a series of acupressure points to deal with specific problem areas like phobias or addictions. It has had highly successful outcomes with PTSD as well. Callahan believed that traumatic memories are trapped within thought fields, and tapping meridians in a specific sequence could allow the traumatic thought to become conscious and allow processing to take place. There have been a series of randomised controlled studies of TFT in Rwandan genocide survivors which indicate significant improvements in several symptoms following TFT. The effects were found to have persistent benefits.

Emotional Freedom Technique: EFT is an offshoot of TFT developed by Gary Craig, a minister and personal trainer. Although both EFT and TFT are quite similar in tapping meridians, there are several differences that make them stand-alone therapies. EFT has a simplified tapping sequence for all emotional problems and has been applied for a variety of conditions. There has been a lot of research into EFT recently. A metaanalysis in 2016 (Sebastian and Nelms) found that EFT was extremely effective in treating PTSD in veterans, with an effect size of 2.96. To give the reader an idea of effect sizes, statisticians consider an effect size of 0.5 to be moderate and 0.8 to be large. One of the studies included in the metaanalysis looked at gene expression in veterans and found that an EFT session regulates 72 different genes. Lasting results were obtained in four to ten sessions.

A 2017 study by Dr. Peta Stapleton, leading EFT researcher at Bond University, Australia, used functional imaging to track fifteen women with obesity before and after four weeks of EFT. She found that the brain rewired itself after tapping, and brain areas which activated hunger in response to certain foods no longer did so after tapping. A review by Dawson Church, leading author and EFT researcher, points out that there are more than 100 clinical trials on the EFT database.

EFT is easily incorporated into clinical practice. Trauma expert Bessel van der Kolk advocates using tapping to complement other therapies in managing PTSD.

Neuro-emotional Technique: NET was developed by Dr. Scott Walker, a chiropractor and applied kinesiologist. He developed NET around the same time that Callahan developed TFT. NET uses psychodynamic concepts as well as kinesiology. Although less known than TFT and EFT, there is some research on NET's beneficial effects in PTSD and ADHD, among other conditions.

II. Reiki:

Reiki was rediscovered in the early 1900s by Japanese theologist, Dr. Mikao Usui. Dr. Usui's intense spiritual practices culminated in his discovery of Reiki, which he passed on to other teachers. Reiki is a simple hands-on healing method during which universal life energy is said to flow from the practitioner's hands to the person receiving treatment. There has been research demonstrating the benefits of Reiki on anxiety reduction, pain, the cardiovascular system, and the immune system. Modest benefits have been demonstrated in depression as well. Reiki has gained immense popularity especially in the United States, with many hospitals offering Reiki as a treatment modality. There are three levels of reiki training, with the master level being the highest (at this level, one can attune other people to Reiki). Although it is a very gentle method of healing, the more one uses it, the more powerfully the energy tends to flow. It would be wrong to judge Reiki only through research on physical and mental ailments, as it heals on many different levels of being, some of which are beyond the scope of this book.

III. Pranic Healing:

Pranic Healing was developed by a spiritual teacher, Master Choa Kok Sui in 1989, and there has been a fair bit of research in a variety of human and cell studies. Dr. Joie Jones has conducted extensive research demonstrating that Pranic healing improved survival of gamma-irradiated cell cultures by 50-90%, irrespective of distance or person providing the treatment.

Another study by Dr. Jones used fMRI imaging to study a subject receiving pranic healing from two experienced practitioners over a specific acupressure point related to vision. The healers' energy stimulated the visual cortex identical to that produced by needle stimulation of the acupoint. Interestingly, the results obtained were the same regardless of whether the healers were near the subject or at a distance. Some other studies have reported improvement on measures of pain, stress, anxiety, nicotine dependence, and accelerated wound healing.

IV. Other Energy therapies:

There are many other energy healing modalities like healing touch, reconnective healing, and Seichim healing which are similar to the ones discussed above. To go into a description of all these modalities is beyond the scope of this book.

Although there is not much research into many of these therapies, it does not mean that they are not effective or valid. As I have mentioned before, there is a dearth of funding into energy healing research. Also, a lot of these healing techniques act on many different levels of being which are not necessarily reflected in standard research studies.

Chapter 14

THE SUPRAMENTAL BODY

INTUITION AND CREATIVITY

"Indeed, it is not intellect, but intuition which advances humanity. Intuition tells man his purpose in this life."

—Albert Einstein

This is the millennium of the brain. We are learning more and more everyday about the two and a half pounds of pink matter we call the seat of our consciousness and our identity. Neuroscientists, with increasingly sophisticated brain imaging techniques, have identified neurological locations that appear to correlate with consciousness, without any conclusive evidence or preferred candidates in the mix.

It is tempting, with the vast increase in our knowledge of neuroscience, to formulate a physical theory of consciousness. Yet, deep thinkers over the ages have not been convinced that consciousness originates in physical structures, as it causes a number of unexplainable paradoxes. A reductionist model of consciousness fails to encapsulate the whole gamut of human experience, including mysticism, spirituality, and creativity—traits which some regard as the very basis of humanity, that which separates us from other living beings. Mystical experiences have been studied and have been found to be associated with a variety of neurochemical, neuroendocrine, and neuroelectrical activities, yet they cannot be proved to be causative of the experiences. Rather, quantum theory points to the primacy of consciousness.

Even more difficult is quantifying and explaining the basis of creativity. Even though human beings have existed on earth for millions of years, technology has advanced by leaps and bounds only in the last few centuries, without any change in the human brain. This burst of creativity seems exponential in its rise and is difficult to explain by generational learning alone.

A now widely cited phenomenon is the 100th monkey phenomenon. Scientists studying a breed of monkeys in Koshima found that a few monkeys learnt to wash sweet potatoes in the stream before eating them and, in a few years, a number of monkeys had learnt to do it. Surprisingly, colonies of monkeys in other islands also started washing their sweet potatoes, even though there was no physical transmission of information from one tribe to another. This points to ways of information sharing beyond the conventional—in a way, it points to the existence of a shared consciousness.

Carl Jung, a renowned psychiatrist, proposed the term "collective unconscious" to a body of knowledge, beliefs, and symbols which are common to all beings of a particular species (in our case, humans) and does not arise from the experience of the individual. Jung believed that all human experience is genetically coded and transferred to successive generations, contributing to the collective unconscious. Contemporary biologist Rupert Sheldrake proposed that this collective information is transmitted across individuals and generations through morphogenetic fields (organising fields that are the blueprint of an individual). Thus, a person can transmit information across time and space, which might explain how people can access knowledge not their own—especially in altered states of consciousness.

Noted psychiatrist Brian Weiss, in his ground-breaking book *Many Lives, Many Masters*(1988), describes a young lady who, when under hypnosis, was able to access and communicate knowledge about him which she had no way of knowing consciously.

Medical mediums have been in existence for centuries, the most celebrated being Edgar Cayce, dubbed "The Sleeping Prophet" because he would put himself in a trance and suggest remedies for a variety of medical conditions. Of course, this was before the time of the pharmaceutical industry boom and a lot of remedies are not what we conventionally use nowadays. Yet, he had surprisingly high rates of success for someone without a medical background.

Nowadays, it is more common to talk about medical intuitives, people with or without medical backgrounds who are able to decipher or diagnose the root cause of a person's medical problem. In 1984, Norman Shealy, a Harvard-trained neurosurgeon, found that a young woman, Caroline Myss, was 93% accurate in her ability to diagnose illness, even from remote distances. She is now a legend in the field of medical intuition, which is gaining recognition.

Today, we have several practitioners of medical intuition, some of whom are intuitive physicians who combine their knowledge of medicine with intuitive knowledge to treat people more effectively. One such physician and intuitive is Dr. Judith Orloff, Professor of Psychiatry at UCLA. In her book, *Second Sight*, Orloff describes her intuitive and psychic experiences, She tried to ignore her experiences for several years before combining it with traditional methods to enhance effectiveness of treatment.

According to Dr. Orloff, intuition is a skill which can be learned by anyone. She cites the example of the Remote Viewing experiments of the U.S. military, who trained regular people to become "psychic spies" by tuning in to their intuition with amazing accuracy.

Intuition is often regarded as our sixth sense, which our left-brained, linear upbringing often tells us to ignore as illogical. Yet, honed correctly and nurtured lovingly, it can be a precise tool at our disposal not only to intuit what is wrong with us, but also to know how to right it. How often have you thought of someone and, right then, you receive a phone call from that person? Have you ever had a niggling feeling of discomfort at the back of your mind just before you got some bad news? We often dismiss such instances as coincidences because they do not happen enough for us to call them otherwise. Those who have highly developed intuitions call them synchronicities.

Intuition is closely linked to creativity, and intuitive people are also highly creative and prolific in their own fields. All the innovation that we enjoy today wouldn't be possible without intuition and creativity, which deserve to be consciously nurtured and cultivated. Intuition not only helps us make better decisions but also improves mental, physical, and emotional well-being.

A common question that people ask is "How do I increase my intuition? And how do I know that it is intuition guiding me?' I have asked myself these questions several times on my journey. I did not consider myself particularly intuitive; I have never had flashes of insight or visions that would convince me to consider myself intuitive. However, I had an epiphany one day and realised that intuition is not limited to seeing. We expect visions and drumroll when we think about intuition, but it can come in different ways for different people. I realised that for me, it often came as an unshakeable feeling. I seem inexorably drawn to a particular path which does not leave room for doubt. I have noticed intuition as the gentle hand that often saves me from taking a path I would regret later. It feels like a power greater than us is gently steering the course of destiny for us. Intuition grows the more we allow ourselves to let go of our rational mind and realise that there is a consciousness greater than our individual mind that is aware of the bigger picture.

As we welcome intuition to stay in our consciousness and steer our ship for us, it allows healing to take place. Hand in hand with intuition comes creativity, which is our true state of being. It is not possible to talk about creativity without being mystical. The urge to create is a primordial urge of all living matter; this urge has led to all evolution. However, the human urge to create moves beyond a mere biological urge to create replicas of ourselves. We desire to be *original* in our creation—this is what separates us from the rest of life and gives us a glimpse of ourselves as creators. In the years that we have been on earth, we have strived to not only create new technology, art, and architecture to make our lives easier and more interesting, but also more beautiful.

I believe that creation is the ultimate healing tool that we have at our disposal. When we create, we can no longer be a victim. Being a creator empowers us in a way that the best therapy cannot. Time and again studies on cancer survivors have shown that survival rates are better in those who actively participate in their treatment, question their healthcare providers, and use tools like creative visualisation along with conventional treatment. This represents a quantum leap from the position of a victim to a creator.

How we create is immaterial. Some create with colour, clay, or stone, some with words, and some with expressions and body movements. All forms of art fundamentally involve a shift from being shaped by our environment to shaping our environment. In doing so, we become masters of the world around us. I believe this is the key to the therapeutic aspects of all art forms. Art therapy and psychodrama have long been known to be beneficial for people with mental illness, but these strategies deserve more attention than they have been given.

The human mind seeks meaning, and all biological therapies and technological advances will remain soulless unless they help people find meaning. Victor Frankl, noted psychiatrist and Auschwitz survivor, proposed in his seminal book, *Man's*

Search for Meaning, that people are primarily driven by a search for meaning in their lives.

We have come a full circle. Despite massive improvements in living standards, life expectancy, and giant leaps in technology, humankind is still plagued by unhappiness, sorrow and mental illness. Healing should not be so much about finding our ideal biological state (although this is undoubtedly important), but instead on finding purpose and meaning in our existence. My vision of a quantum psychiatrist is one who helps people find meaning while optimising their physical, emotional, mental and spiritual state.

Chapter 15

THROUGH THE LOOKING GLASS

QUANTUM PSYCHIATRY IN ACTION

"Learn from yesterday, live for today, hope for tomorrow. The important thing is not to stop questioning."

—Albert Einstein

So, how can quantum psychiatry heal someone? In the following hypothetical vignette, I draw from my own experience with clients to demonstrate, step-by-step, how the quantum psychiatry model can help heal clients who have not responded to conventional treatments.

Leila is a thirty-four-year-old mother of two children who had a recent deterioration in her mental health. Growing up, she experienced abandonment and neglect by her mother, who left her with her father when she was three years old. Leila was raised by her stepmother, who discriminated between her and her own children. Leila struggled with anxiety during her teenage years and resorted to cutting herself to help cope with overwhelming emotions. She saw psychologists and learnt the basic cognitive techniques, but they never seemed to help when she was in the throes of an anxiety attack. As an adult, she was insecure in her relationship, and worried that her husband would leave her. However, she managed to function and worked full time in an administrative position.

Things came to a head when her father passed away and, at the same time, she was made redundant at work. Leila started having severe panic attacks, and suicidal thoughts became a regular part of her life. Her eating was out of control and she began restricting her calories, resulting in significant weight loss. She tried several antidepressant medications but nothing seemed to work. Finally she saw a quantum psychiatrist, who helped unpackage her problems like peeling the layers of an onion.

The first step was to address her "here and now" symptoms of depression and anxiety. In addition to basic blood work, Leila underwent pharmacogenomic testing, which indicated that she was a fast metabolizer of the antidepressant she was currently on. She had a quantitative EEG which provided valuable information on the class of medication she was likely to respond to; her antidepressant was then changed, in alignment with the pharmacogenomic and QEEG report.

Next, the psychiatrist explained to Leila how her past experience of abandonment and neglect at an early age had affected her limbic system—the emotional brain, which develops before the neocortex (logical brain) develops. She now understood why, despite years of cognitive therapy, her anxiety would still throw her off: since the limbic system develops when we are preverbal, talk therapy could not reach the limbic brain. Leila began to have sessions of neurofeedback to regulate her limbic system, which was perpetually in fight or flight mode. She also learnt that traumatic memories are not just encoded in her brain, but also in her body. She began sessions of yoga and pranayama, which helped her become grounded and comfortable in her own body.

As she progressed, spontaneous memories of traumatic events which had happened when she was a child started to resurface. Although it was easier to handle them now, Leila wanted to delve deeper into these memories. Her psychologist started EMDR in conjunction with neurofeedback to help Leila process those memories. At the same time, she learnt "tapping" or Emotional Freedom Technique, with positive effects not only on her memories, but also her energy and vitality.

Like many other people before her, Leila often asked the question, "Why me?" Her quantum psychiatrist encouraged her to reframe and ask instead, "What did I learn from this experience, and how can I move forward?" Simply changing the question shifted Leila's consciousness from being a victim to being a creator. She began to meditate to develop a deeper connection with her spiritual self. She began to make the connection between her past experiences and current insecurities and worked on strengthening her root chakra. She understood now that although she was not happy at her work, she hung in there because it represented security. As she became more rooted to her own sense of self, she became more creative. She started painting again, something she had not done for several years. Her canvases were now splashed with colour and meaning, as was her life. Although offered another administrative position, she decided not to accept it but to exhibit her paintings professionally in a gallery instead. Her exhibition was a huge success and she received accolades for her work.

Leila's story is not unique. Day in and day out, I listen to stories of violence, hatred, abandonment and sorrow. The physical bodies change, the contexts change, but the emotions remain the same.

Countless times, I have been asked by troubled patients, "Why me?" For a long time, I answered according to my conventional training, parrot-like: "You have a genetic predisposition due to a strong family history, and this, coupled with the abandonment you faced in childhood, predisposes you to anxiety. Your loss and current redundancy has created a crisis as it retriggered feelings of abandonment." This is what a psychiatric formulation looks like.

Then, suddenly, it hit me between the eyes. This is not what people want to know. They are seeking to *find* meaning in their suffering; they need to know why they had to go through the experience they did. As a quantum psychiatrist, I can encourage them to *give* meaning to their suffering, moving them from a state of victimhood to a state of creation. This is the role I envisage for the future quantum psychiatrist—not just an expert in a range of diagnostic and therapeutic techniques, but also a guide and a mentor who nudges people along to reconnect with their quantum selves.

If you are someone who has had traumatic or negative life experiences for a long time, or someone who has been with the black dog of depression for so long that it almost feels like a friend, you might find it hard to believe that change is possible. Yet, this is my message to you: change is possible. People have overcome immense adversities and moved to more fulfilling lives through the techniques outlined in this book. At our core, we are all quantum beings, and we all exist in the realm of possibility. Whatever experiences you might have had in the past, you can choose not to let it determine the rest of your future. I raise a toast to your glorious future.

Part 3

BACK TO THE FUTURE

Chapter 16

FROM HUMAN BEINGS TO QUANTUM BEINGS

"A human being is a part of the whole called by us universe, a part limited in time and space. He experiences himself, his thoughts and feeling as something separated from the rest, a kind of optical delusion of his consciousness. This delusion is a kind of prison for us, restricting us to our personal desires and to affection for a few persons nearest to us. Our task must be to free ourselves from this prison by widening our circle of compassion to embrace all living creatures and the whole of nature in its beauty."

—Albert Einstein

We are all individuations in a quantum field of possibility. We might feel alienated or separated from others, but we can catch glimpses of the quantum field of possibility through meditation and intuition. The quantum field of possibility is the collective consciousness we tap into during dreams and spiritual experiences. We are both the observer and the observed, in a tangled hierarchy. There exists in the quantum field many alternate possibilities, and when we choose to pay attention to one particular possibility, it collapses into reality. Although this might seem immutable, it is still a part of the quantum field. Focusing on an alternate possibility will result in a quantum shift, which then becomes reality. This is not a fairy tale—it is no different from the position of an electron, which collapses into a particular position when observed.

The concept of a quantum field of possibility explains how people experience spontaneous healing: they have now chosen to focus on an alternative reality in the quantum field. This is not a forcing of the consciousness to change direction, but a total shift of attention to a different place.

The question is: How do we experience this healing consciousness? This is in fact part of a larger question of how to move from existing as a human being to a quantum being. Meditate and pay attention to your dreams and intuition. Become aware of yourself as a part of the quantum field, individuated but not separated from the field. Consciousness pervades the quantum field, and we all share this collective consciousness. Our thoughts and actions influence this consciousness as the consciousness influences us. As we observe the myriad of possibilities that exist in this field, we can choose to focus on one particular possibility in order to collapse it into reality. Meditation brings this process under conscious control.

Once we recognise the quantum field and our place in it, we become increasingly aware of the pervasive energy around us. This is the living, conscious, dynamic energy swirling around the cosmos. Call it "chi" or "prana" or "universal energy"—it is a formidable force that cannot be exploited or commanded, but only invited to be a part of your life, if and when you are ready.

The journey might be long, but it is immensely rewarding and liberating. Be assured that when you are ready to embrace your quantum self, you will be guided—through your dreams, intuitions, synchronicities, and many other ways that will leave no room for doubt.

Chapter 17

GEN Z OR GEN Q?

"If you want your children to be intelligent, read them fairy tales. If you want them to be more intelligent, read them more fairy tales."

—Albert Einstein

The children of today, also called Gen Z, will determine the future of the earth. After generations who have suffered the ravages of war, poverty, exploitation, and abuse, humanity is finally evolving to be a more tolerant species. When I see today's children, I see hope. Although innocent, they are often mature beyond their years. They are growing up in an age of multiculturalism, an age of activism. I see them more accepting of different skin colours, accents, and languages. I see them voice concerns for the environment and take up the cause of the voiceless. They are more tolerant of different religions and cultural identities and celebrate happily with each other. They are accepting of people of different genders, or even no gender. It seems to me that dichotomies are slowly being replaced by spectrums. Our children are truly global citizens and I hope they are able to see a world free from the cruelties of our past generations.

I hope for quantum psychiatry to start healing the wounds of our generation. As we heal, we will create a more nurturing environment for our children and put an end to the intergenerational transmission of trauma. If there is one thing you can give your children, give them the freedom to dream. If there is one thing that you can help your children with, help them love themselves. If there is one thing you can teach your children, teach them how to meditate. For in the stillness of the mind, the heart soars beyond all duality and experiences true freedom. Let us free our next Generation, the Quantum Generation.

Appendix

QUANTUM MEDITATIONS

"Don't listen to the person who has the answers; listen to the person who has the questions."

—Albert Einstein

I have discussed a range of interventions in this book, but I cannot over-emphasise the power of meditation. There have been numerous studies on the effect of meditation on brain waves and physiology. Imagine if I told you that it is possible to improve not just your mental health, but also your general health, well-being, and immunity with a treatment—and it is completely free! If meditation came in a bottle, it would be called a miracle drug.

However, many people find it difficult to develop a meditation practice for a variety of reasons, some of which I outline below:

Difficulty in persisting with techniques which emphasise an empty mind.

A perception that meditation is esoteric and spiritual and not for the scientifically minded

Some people believe that it conflicts with their religious ideals.

For those with a history of trauma, feeling unsafe with their eyes closed.

Feeling overwhelmed.

Thoughts wandering during sessions.

The following meditations are written to encourage all such readers to start a regular meditation practice. They are available as mp3 recordings free to download with the book. The meditations move step-by-step through the chakras, from the root to the crown. They have been specially recorded with the specific sound frequency of each chakra to help in its activation. Ideally, listen to a particular meditation as many times as needed, till you feel ready to move on to the next meditation. They are designed to help open your awareness and access higher states of consciousness. I hope they are just the beginning of your journey into quantum consciousness.

Meditation 1

FEELING SAFE

CONNECTING TO THE ROOT CHAKRA

Close your eyes and breathe slowly, in and out, in and out. Bring your awareness to your breath, as it moves in and out of your nostrils. This breath nourishes and nurtures you gently. It is like an anchor for your mind, allowing you to slow down and drop anchor when emotions make the mind turbulent. As you breathe in, imagine the breath drop like an anchor, down through your throat, through your chest, through your abdomen, right down to your hips and your feet. As you breathe in and out, imagine this anchor getting wider and stronger. Continue making your anchor stronger.

Now, I want you to bring your attention to your lower body. Notice the surface you are sitting on. Imagine this surface to be a rock, where you can drop your anchor. This is your own personal rock, your safe place, inaccessible to anyone else. Visualise this rock in detail. Picture any nooks or crannies it might have. Is the surface smooth? Is it warm? Now imagine going inside this rock. It seems solid, but it is actually buzzing with atoms and electrons. Imagine this buzzing energy of the rock spread to your feet, and then your hips. Visualise this buzzing energy as a red light moving up your feet to your hips. This energy grounds you and makes you feel safe. Stay with this energy as long as you can. Allow it to nourish you and empower you.

Allow this red energy to stay with you. It helps you recognise that you are your own person, walking in your own power. As you slowly open your eyes, remember that you can always anchor to your rock with your breath and draw on this energy to feel safe and grounded on this earth and in this physical body.

Meditation 2

COSMIC CREATIVITY

CONNECTING TO THE SACRAL CHAKRA

Close your eyes and gently start breathing in and out, in and out. Bring your attention to your breath as you gently watch the ebb and flow of your breath. Do not try to control it, just be with it.

You will notice after a few breaths that your breath starts following your awareness. Gently direct your awareness to your spinal column and imagine a column of light flow down from your crown down to your hips. (Pause.) Imagine a ball of orange light forming in the centre of your hips. As it grows larger, it glows brighter and starts spinning, at first slowly, and gradually speeding up, till it is like a vortex. As it spins, it starts releasing incredible energy into your body and all around you. See the sparks of energy flashing all around you, filling every cell of your body with strength and purpose.

This is the creative energy stored at the base of your spine. The sparks represent cosmic or quantum creativity, which is now moving into every cell of your body, igniting your personal creativity. You realise that you have released the wellspring of creativity within the core of your being. You recognise intuitively that you are an inherently creative being. Creativity is ingrained in your biology and in your destiny. Every day, you create millions of cells within your body. You manufacture an array of thoughts, intentions, and actions out of seeming nothingness, and your thoughts in turn create your future.

As you tap into this orange light, this wellspring of creativity, you become more conscious of this process of creation. You recognise your power as a creator: of your cells, of your hormones, of your chemicals, and your thoughts. Imbibe the orange glow into all your cells and recognise that you are a creator.

Allow the orange energy to stay with you. Now, when you are ready, slowly open your eyes. As you move into everyday awareness, you will carry with you the spark of creativity which will ignite your passion for life henceforth.

Meditation 3

WHO AM I?

CONNECTING TO THE SOLAR PLEXUS

Close your eyes and start breathing gently, in and out, in and out, like the waves upon the sand. Relax every part of your body so that it goes limp as you bring your awareness inside yourself. Now, we are going to find our true identity. Watch the thoughts come and go like waves upon sand and observe them calming down. The waves are smaller, gentler, quieter, as if they can understand the power of silence. As the silence grows, all you hear is buzzing—the buzzing of the energy of earth, the energy of your body and mind. Just pure energy. And in this buzzing silence, a question comes to you: Who am I?

Note the first response that comes. Maybe plumber, pharmacist, secretary, homemaker? Observe this, and notice that this is just a layer covering who you are. Peel this layer off and ask the question again: Who am I?

What is the answer you get this time? Perhaps it is a bit closer to your heart. Mother, son, friend? But this again is a role you play, another layer covering who you are. Peel this layer off, and ask the question again: Who am I?

Listen to the answer this time. Perhaps the answer is more abstract this time: artist, dreamer, a kind person? Again, these are qualities that you possess or things you like to do, but not your true identity. Peel this layer off as well, and ask the question again: Who am I?

Maybe you identify with your body, or your mind, or other attributes or possessions. Note that these are simply attributes or possessions, not your true identity. Peel this layer off as well and ask the question: Who am I? Note the answers as you peel off layer after layer, veil after veil.

Who are you? You are beyond your profession, your roles, your likes, your body, your mind, your thoughts. Perhaps some of the answers you come up with are these: Observer. Consciousness. Light. Source. Soul. Spirit. I am.

Whatever you choose to call it, how does it make you feel? Free, limitless, boundless, dispassionate, pure love, pure light? However you choose to interpret this experience, it has profoundly affected you at a fundamental level. As you gradually come back to your mind and body and open your eyes, carry with you this awareness of your true self in your everyday life.

Meditation 4

THE SOURCE WITHIN

CONNECTING TO THE HEART CHAKRA

Close your eyes and start breathing gently in and out. Gently bring your awareness to your breath as it rhythmically moves in and out.... in and out, like the waves of the ocean. Now, I want you to bring your awareness to your heart. Imagine that you are breathing through your heart—in and out, in and out. Now, I want you to picture the most beautiful golden light and imagine that you are breathing in this golden light through your heart, in and out, in and out. See the brilliant light swirling within your chest cavity as it fills your heart with fresh energy and love. Keep breathing this golden light for a while.

Now, I want you to visualise someone or something in your life that you appreciate. It might be a person, a pet, a plant, anything that you appreciate. Visualise this person or thing in your heart, within the golden light, and feel the appreciation spreading through your chest and heart. Notice the sensation this feeling brings with it. Is it warm and fuzzy, like the summer sunshine? Is it tingling, like ice on your fingertips? Is it an inner glow, like the gentle moonlight at night? Sit with this feeling for a while.

Now, allow this feeling to start expanding. Let it flow, like wisps of clouds, into every corner of your being. Feel it move into your arms, your abdomen, your hips. Feel it trickling down your legs to your feet. Feel it moving up into your throat, like a warm cup of tea, and up into your head cavity. Feel this gentle energy behind your eyes. Let your body soak up this feeling of appreciation. It feels like water upon parched soil. Let the feeling swirl around you and within you, nurturing you. Sit with this feeling for a while.

You have tapped into the source of love, which is gentle and unconditional and demands nothing of you. Its warm glow slowly heals all emotional wounds and feelings of loss or lack, as light heals darkness. It is for everyone, yet it is for you alone. It connects you to all that is around you. Let this feeling rest behind your eyeballs and imagine seeing through those eyes. It allows you to see the world with fresh eyes, and appreciate the beautiful world we live in. Can you see the lush green trees, the rushing water in the ocean, the sweet song of birds up in the trees? This world was made for you to live in and appreciate. Begin to notice all the wonders of nature. Thank Nature for her gifts.

Now, with an awareness of this feeling in your heart, in your body, and behind your eyes, slowly open your eyes. Feel free to come back to this meditation as often as you like, and reconnect to this healing energy of the Source within.

Meditation 5

OWNING YOUR STORY

CONNECTING TO THE THROAT CHAKRA

Close your eyes and begin to breathe slowly and gently, in and out, in and out. Bring your awareness to your breath as it flows in and out of your nostrils. Imagine the breath moving into your throat. As it moves in, it transforms into a brilliant blue light in the centre of your throat. Focus on the blue light for a while. This light carries your truth, your story. What does it tell you? As you look at this blue light, ask yourself: are you completely honest with yourself? Are you being true to who you really are? Take a moment to ponder these questions.

Now, imagine the light getting stronger and more powerful as you stand in front of a mirror. There is only one person in this world who knows who you truly are, and that person is staring you in the eye. This person has seen it all—your trials and tribulations, your joys and victories, your shame and embarrassment. This person knows where you are coming from and is someone you can tell your story to. There is no need for any mask, any bravado, or any pretence in front of this person; you can truly be free to express who you are. Tell this person who you are and who you wish to be.

Now, the brilliant blue ball of light expands and glows more intensely, and as it does so, so does its reflection in the mirror. Both balls expand to the point that they begin to merge into each other. See them merging together, as you begin to accept your story and who you are.

The blue balls of light have now merged and enveloped your whole being and your reflection. This is your life, and your story: this is who you are. Once you own your story, you are ready to move forward to wherever you want to go. See the blue light with your story envelop your being.

Now, when you are ready, gently open your eyes, with an awareness of authenticity. You may choose to share your story with others, or you may choose to share it only with yourself—but you have now accepted it, and are ready to move forward.

Meditation 6

EMBRACING THE WAVE OF QUANTUM POSSIBILITY

CONNECTING TO THE THIRD EYE

Close your eyes and take some deep breaths in and out, in and out. Bring your awareness to your breath. As you breathe in through your nostrils, imagine the breath going upwards towards the top of your head. As you breathe out, imagine the breath travelling down from the top of your head and out through your nostrils. Keep doing this for a while.

Now, I want you to rest your awareness on your brow, between your eyes. Imagine your breath accumulating there as a ball of light which keeps expanding. As it expands, visualise another ball of light just on top of your head, but outside of you. This ball of light is the wave of possibility. It contains all possible past and future scenarios of your life. The ball of light within your head represents your current state of consciousness. Now, imagine the ball of light above your head, the wave of possibility, starting to slowly move down, down, down, till it meets the light within your head, your consciousness. Witness both these balls of light slowly merging together. As they do so, there is a single ball of light which shines brighter and starts expanding, more and more, until it fills your whole head cavity. Imagine it growing larger and larger.

Have a look within this ball. Do you see glimpses of your current life the way it is? Now look again. The wave of possibility contains all possible versions of your life. What do you choose to focus on? Where would you like your life to move from this point forward? Focus on the possibility that appeals to you and resonates with you the most. Imagine this possibility to the fullest.

Now, imagine this possibility separating from the ball of light and forming its own little ball of light. Now the rest of the wave of possibility moves back up through the top of your head till it melts into the universal consciousness. The possibility you have chosen is now within your third eye as your new reality. Relish the new reality you have chosen for a while.

Now, when you are ready, slowly open your eyes, with an awareness that you have chosen a new reality. Come back to this meditation whenever you want, to reinforce this new reality, or to choose a new reality.

Meditation 7

QUANTUM EXISTENCE

CONNECTING TO THE CROWN CHAKRA

Close your eyes and sit comfortably, either cross-legged or on a chair. Breathe gently in and out…in and out. Feel your entire body relax and become limp, like a rag doll. Focus your attention on your breath and the music in the background, going deeper and deeper into your awareness and into your body.

Now, I want you to imagine yourself, the observer, shrinking gradually, becoming smaller and smaller. As you become smaller, notice where your awareness takes you inside your body. Are you in your brain, at the back of your eyes, or somewhere in your heart or belly? Wherever you are, imagine yourself shrinking to the size of a cell. Observe yourself within this cell and see what you observe. Perhaps you can see the nucleus, or the mitochondria floating around? Notice how they look as you start shrinking again. You are now down to the size of a tiny ribosome, and even the cell looks like a giant room to you.

Now, you are shrinking down further and further till you are the size of the molecules in the cell. Notice the individual molecules that make up the giant structures around you. You can see molecules entering and exiting the cell through the membrane, and you can now yourself come in and out of the cell and the nucleus at will.

Now, you are shrinking down further again, even smaller than a molecule. You can see the individual atoms that make up a molecule. Perhaps you can see a water molecule, which now looks so big to you. You are now smaller than an atom.

You witness the dance of the cosmos in the atom you are in. The nucleus, like a star, around which the electrons dance around, jumping from one axis to another. You watch with awe as electrons disappear from one place, only to appear in another instantaneously. You hear the buzzing of the cosmos within the atom, as the electrons flit around. They are everywhere and nowhere at the same time.

Now, you feel a tremendous energy propel you outwards. You shoot out of the atom, out of the molecule, out of the membrane of the cell, out of the organ, and out of the physical body. But you are still the size of an electron, and you can see the millions of electrons zapping around millions of nuclei, like the galaxies of the universe. As you observe, you see them not just as electrons, but as energy, and you can see each of their energy fields combine to form an energy field around the physical body, extending beyond the limits of the body. And you realise that you are not just physical, but a bundle of energy at the same time that extends beyond your physical body. And it is no longer a paradox, because you have experienced it first-hand.

You move back into your body, into the cell you were in, and you can see the dance of energy around you. This energy is self-organising and self-directing and never-tiring. Sit in this energy for a moment and soak it up.

Now, you find yourself growing bigger gradually. You are the size of a molecule, then a ribosome, then a nucleus, and you keep growing and expanding, till you are back where you belong. But where do you belong? You are pure consciousness, you belong everywhere that you choose to belong, from the smallest subatomic particle to the limitlessness of the ever-expanding universe.

Sit with this awareness that you have now experienced and gradually allow yourself to come back to your body and mind, as you open your eyes. Quantum knowledge has now been transformed into Quantum knowing, which will stay with you from this point onwards.

BIBLIOGRAPHY AND SUGGESTED READING

Introduction
The Journey Begins

Chopra, Deepak. 1989. *Quantum healing : exploring the frontiers of mind/ body medicine*: Bantam.

Dyer, Wayne W. 2001. *Real magic : creating miracles in everyday life*. New York: Quill.

Isherwood, Christopher. *Vedanta for the western world*: [S.l.] : Allen & Unwin, 1951.

Morris, J.J. 1999. *Reiki: Hands that heal.* Boston: Weiser Books.

Diagnostic and statistical manual of mental disorders : DSM-5. Fifth edition. ed.

PART 1: THE THEORIES SHAPING QUANTUM PSYCHIATRY

Chapter 1
Tinker, Tailor, Soldier, Sailor

Goswami, Amit. 2017. *The everything answer book : how quantum science explains love, death, and the meaning of life*. Charlottesville, VA: Hampton Roads.

Gawain, Shakti. 2008. *Creative visualization : use the power of your imagination to create what you want in your life*. 30th anniversary ed. Novato, Calif.: Nataraj Pub.

Chapter 2
Adventures in Wonderland: Quantum Physics and the Brain

-----1979 January 1, Brain Mind Bulletin, Volume 4, Number 4, 'Consciousness is the primary reality' Nobel physicist tells N.Y. symposium, Start Page 3, Quote Page 3, Published by Interface Press, Los Angeles, California.

Goswami, Amit, Richard E. Reed, and Maggie Goswami. 1993. *The self-aware universe : how consciousness creates the material world*. London: Simon & Schuster.

Von Neumann, John. 1996. *Mathematical foundations of quantum mechanics*. Princeton ; Chichester: Princeton University Press.

Penrose, Roger. 1989. *The emperor's new mind : concerning computers, minds, and the laws of physics*. Oxford: Oxford University Press.

Goswami, Amit. 2004. *The quantum doctor : a physicist's guide to health and healing*. Charlottesville, VA: Hampton Roads Pub.

Chapter 3
Spooky Action at a distance: Signal-less communication

--- EPR paradox:
https://en.wikipedia.org/wiki/EPR_paradox Accessed 21 May 2020

Chapter 4
The Guard dog, the Elephant and the Wise Owl: The Neuroscience of Mental Illness

Heisenberg, Werner. 1971. *Physics and beyond encounters and conversations*. New York: Harper and Row.

Robbins, Jim. 2008. *A symphony in the brain : the evolution of the new brain wave biofeedback*. Rev. ed. ed. New York: Grove.

Rizzolatti, G., L. Fadiga, L. Fogassi, and V. Gallese. 1999. "Resonance behaviors and mirror neurons." *Arch Ital Biol* 137 (2-3):85-100.

Chapter 5
Glia and Einstein's Brain

García-Cáceres, C., C. Quarta, L. Varela, Y. Gao, T. Gruber, B. Legutko, M. Jastroch, P. Johansson, J. Ninkovic, C. X. Yi, O. Le Thuc, K. Szigeti-Buck, W. Cai, C. W. Meyer, P. T. Pfluger, A. M. Fernandez, S. Luquet, S. C. Woods, I. Torres-Alemán, C. R. Kahn, M. Götz, T. L. Horvath, and M. H. Tschöp. 2016. "Astrocytic Insulin Signaling Couples Brain Glucose Uptake with Nutrient Availability." *Cell* 166 (4):867-880. doi: 10.1016/j.cell.2016.07.028.

Bonnefil, V., K. Dietz, M. Amatruda, M. Wentling, A. V. Aubry, J. L. Dupree, G. Temple, H. J. Park, N. S. Burghardt, P. Casaccia, and J. Liu. 2019. "Region-specific myelin differences define behavioral consequences of chronic social defeat stress in mice." *Elife* 8. doi: 10.7554/eLife.40855.

Zhou, X., Q. Xiao, L. Xie, F. Yang, L. Wang, and J. Tu. 2019. "Astrocyte, a Promising Target for Mood Disorder

Interventions." *Front Mol Neurosci* 12:136. doi: 10.3389/fnmol.2019.00136.

Koob, Andrew. 2009. *The root of thought : unlocking glia--the brain cell that will help us sharpen our wits, heal injury, and treat brain disease.* Upper Saddle River, N.J.: Financial Times/Prentice Hall ; London : Pearson Education [distributor].

Chapter 6
The seat of the soul: The Pineal gland

Strassman, Rick. 2000. *DMT : the spirit molecule : a doctor's revolutionary research into the biology of near-death and mystical experiences.* Rochester, Vt.: Park Street Press.

Bastos, M. A. V., P. R. H. Oliveira Bastos, R. B. Portella, L. F. G. Soares, R. B. Conde, P. M. F. Rodrigues, and G. Lucchetti. 2019. "Pineal gland and schizophrenia: A systematic review and meta-analysis." *Psychoneuroendocrinology* 104:100-114. doi: 10.1016/j.psyneuen.2019.02.024.

Fındıklı, E., M. F. Inci, M. Gökçe, H. A. Fındıklı, H. Altun, and M. F. Karaaslan. 2015. "Pineal gland volume in schizophrenia and mood disorders." *Psychiatr Danub* 27 (2):153-8.

Bumb, J. M., D. Mier, I. Noelte, M. Schredl, P. Kirsch, O. Hennig, L. Liebrich, S. Fenske, B. Alm, C. Sauer, F. M.

Leweke, and E. Sobanski. 2016. "Associations of pineal volume, chronotype and symptom severity in adults with attention deficit hyperactivity disorder and healthy controls." *Eur Neuropsychopharmacol* 26 (7):1119-26. doi: 10.1016/j.euroneuro.2016.03.016.

Song, J. 2019. "Pineal gland dysfunction in Alzheimer's disease: relationship with the immune-pineal axis, sleep disturbance, and neurogenesis." *Mol Neurodegener* 14 (1):28. doi: 10.1186/s13024-019-0330-8.

Xu C, Wang L, Tan Y, Li Q. 2001. Endonasal low energy He-Ne laser treatment of insomnia. Qian Wei J Med & Pharm. 18(5): 337-338 (in Chinese)

Chapter 7
Ball of Light: The Human Energy Field

Ross, C. L. 2019. "Energy Medicine: Current Status and Future Perspectives." *Glob Adv Health Med* 8:2164956119831221. doi: 10.1177/2164956119831221.

Burr, Harold Saxton. 1972. *The fields of life : our links with the universe*. New York: Ballantyne Books.

Becker, Robert O., and Gary Selden. 1985. *The Body Electric : electromagnetism and the foundation of life*. 1st Quill ed. New York: Quill.

Gurwitsch, A. A. 1988. "A historical review of the problem of mitogenetic radiation." *Experientia* 44 (7):545-50. doi: 10.1007/BF01953301.

Swanson, Claude. 2011. *Life Force, The Scientific Basis: Breakthrough Physics of Energy Medicine, Healing, Chi and Quantum Consciousness.* 2nd ed. II vols. Vol. II, *The Synchronized Universe*: Poseidia Press.

Sheldrake, Rupert. 1981. *A new science of life : the hypothesis of formative causation.* London: Blond & Briggs.

Watson, Lyall. 1987. *Lifetide.* [Sevenoaks]: Sceptre.

Jung, C. G. 1969. *The archetypes and the collective unconscious.* 2nd ed. ed. [S.l.]: Routledge & Kegan Paul.

Chapter 8
Energy vortices of the body: The Chakras

Korotkov, K. 2004. *Measuring energy field : state-of-the-science.* Fair Lawn, N.J.: Backbone ; [Lancaster : Gazelle].

Pert, Candace B. 1997. *Molecules of emotion : why you feel the way you feel.* London: Simon & Schuster, 1998.

Erikson, Erik H. 1959. *Identity and the life cycle : Selected papers.* [S.l.]: [s.n.].

Maslow, Abraham H., and Richard Lowry. 1999. *Toward a psychology of being*. 3rd ed. ed. New York ; Chichester: Wiley.

Sheldrake, Rupert. 2009. *Morphic resonance : the nature of formative causation*. 4th, rev. and expanded U.S. ed. ed. Rochester, Vt.: Park Street Press.

Goswami, Amit. 1994. *Science within consciousness : developing a science based on the primacy of consciousness*. Sausalito, Calif.: Institute of Noetic Sciences in partnership with Fetzer Institute.

Azeemi, S. T., and S. M. Raza. 2005. "A critical analysis of chromotherapy and its scientific evolution." *Evid Based Complement Alternat Med* 2 (4):481-8. doi: 10.1093/ecam/neh137

Chapter 9
Rivers of energy: The Nadis or Meridians

Stefanov, M., M. Potroz, J. Kim, J. Lim, R. Cha, and M. H. Nam. 2013. "The primo vascular system as a new anatomical system." *J Acupunct Meridian Stud* 6 (6):331-8. doi: 10.1016/j.jams.2013.10.001.

Rahnama, M., J. A. Tuszynski, I. Bókkon, M. Cifra, P. Sardar, and V. Salari. 2011. "Emission of mitochondrial biophotons and their effect on electrical activity of membrane via microtubules." *J Integr Neurosci* 10 (1):65-88. doi: 10.1142/S0219635211002622.

Saoji, A. A., B. R. Raghavendra, and N. K. Manjunath. 2019. "Effects of yogic breath regulation: A narrative review of scientific evidence." *J Ayurveda Integr Med* 10 (1):50-58. doi: 10.1016/j.jaim.2017.07.008.

Schore, Allan N. author Ucla David Geffen School of Medicine. *Right Brain Psychotherapy (Norton Series on Interpersonal Neurobiology)*.

Marshall, R. S., A. Basilakos, T. Williams, and K. Love-Myers. 2014. "Exploring the benefits of unilateral nostril breathing practice post-stroke: attention, language, spatial abilities, depression, and anxiety." *J Altern Complement Med* 20 (3):185-94. doi: 10.1089/acm.2013.0019.

PART 2: QUANTUM LEVELS OF HEALING

Chapter 10
The Physical body

Longo, Robert. 2018. *A consumer's guide to understanding QEEG brain mapping and neurofeedback training*. iUniverse.

Doidge, Norman. 2007. *The brain that changes itself : stories of personal triumph from the frontiers of brain science.* New York: Viking.

Doidge, Norman. 2015. *The brain's way of healing : stories of remarkable recoveries and discoveries.*

Merzenich, M. 2013. *Soft-Wired: How the new science of brain plasticity can change your life.* 2nd ed: Parnassus Publishing.

Chi, R. P., and A. W. Snyder. 2012. "Brain stimulation enables the solution of an inherently difficult problem." *Neurosci Lett* 515 (2):121-4. doi: 10.1016/j.neulet.2012.03.012.

Shekelle, P., I. Cook, I. M. Miake-Lye, S. Mak, M. S. Booth, R. Shanman, and J. M. Beroes. 2018. "The Effectiveness and Risks of Cranial Electrical Stimulation for the Treatment of Pain, Depression, Anxiety, PTSD, and Insomnia: A Systematic Review." In. *Evidence-based Synthesis Program* Department of Veterans Affairs, Washington DC

Cimpianu, C. L., W. Strube, P. Falkai, U. Palm, and A. Hasan. 2017. "Vagus nerve stimulation in psychiatry: a systematic review of the available evidence." *J Neural Transm (Vienna)* 124 (1):145-158. doi: 10.1007/s00702-016-1642-2.

Porges, Stephen W. 2011. *The polyvagal theory : neurophysiological foundations of emotions, attachment, communication, and self-regulation.* 1st ed. ed. New York ; London: W.W. Norton.

Lindenfeld, G. 2015. *The twenty-minute trauma fix: New brain science supports healing of PTSD.* 1st ed: CreateSpace Independent Publishing Platform.

Siever, Dave. 2003. "Audio-Visual Entrainment: History and Physiological Mechanisms." *Biofeedback Magazine* 31 (2):1-16.

Zomorrodi, R., G. Loheswaran, A. Pushparaj, and L. Lim. 2019. "Pulsed Near Infrared Transcranial and Intranasal Photobiomodulation Significantly Modulates Neural Oscillations: a pilot exploratory study." *Sci Rep* 9 (1):6309. doi: 10.1038/s41598-019-42693-x.

Rohan, M. L., R. T. Yamamoto, C. T. Ravichandran, K. R. Cayetano, O. G. Morales, D. P. Olson, G. Vitaliano, S. M. Paul, and B. M. Cohen. 2014. "Rapid mood-elevating effects of low field magnetic stimulation in depression." *Biol Psychiatry* 76 (3):186-93. doi: 10.1016/j.biopsych.2013.10.024.

Martiny, K., M. Lunde, and P. Bech. 2010. "Transcranial low voltage pulsed electromagnetic fields in patients with treatment-resistant depression." *Biol Psychiatry* 68 (2):163-9. doi: 10.1016/j.biopsych.2010.02.017.

Straasø, B., L. Lauritzen, M. Lunde, M. Vinberg, L. Lindberg, E. R. Larsen, S. Dissing, and P. Bech. 2014. "Dose-remission of pulsating electromagnetic fields as augmentation in therapy-resistant depression: a randomized, double-blind controlled study." *Acta Neuropsychiatr* 26 (5):272-9. doi: 10.1017/neu.2014.5.

Chapter 11
The Mental body

Burns, David D. 1999. *Feeling good : the new mood therapy*. New York: Avon.

Chapter 12
The Emotional body

Van der Kolk, Bessel A. 2014. *The body keeps the score : mind, brain and body in the transformation of trauma*. Penguin books.

van der Kolk, B. A., H. Hodgdon, M. Gapen, R. Musicaro, M. K. Suvak, E. Hamlin, and J. Spinazzola. 2016. "A Randomized Controlled Study of Neurofeedback for Chronic PTSD." *PLoS One* 11 (12):e0166752. doi: 10.1371/journal.pone.0166752.

Khan, A. M., S. Dar, R. Ahmed, R. Bachu, M. Adnan, and V. P. Kotapati. 2018. "Cognitive Behavioral Therapy versus Eye Movement Desensitization and Reprocessing in Patients with Post-traumatic Stress Disorder: Systematic Review and Meta-analysis of Randomized Clinical Trials." *Cureus* 10 (9):e3250. doi: 10.7759/cureus.3250.

Hildebrand, A, Grand D, and Stemmler M. 2017. "Brainspotting – the efficacy of a new therapy approach for the treatment of Posttraumatic Stress Disorder in comparison to Eye Movement Desensitization and Reprocessing." *Mediterranean Journal of Clinical Psychology* 5 (1).

"Quick coherence technique." https://www.heartmath.org/resources/heartmath-tools/quick-coherence-technique-for-adults/ accessed 20 May 2020.

Lloyd, A., D. Brett, and K. Wesnes. 2010. "Coherence training in children with attention-deficit hyperactivity disorder: cognitive functions and behavioral changes." *Altern Ther Health Med* 16 (4):34-42.

McCraty, R., M. Atkinson, D. Tomasino, J. Goelitz, and H. N. Mayrovitz. 1999. "The impact of an emotional self-management skills course on psychosocial functioning and autonomic recovery to stress in middle school children." *Integr Physiol Behav Sci* 34 (4):246-68. doi: 10.1007/BF02688693.

Chapter 13
The Energy body

Zimmerman, J. 1990. "Laying-on-of-hands healing and therapeutic touch:A testable theory." *BEMI Currents, Journal of the Bio-Electro-Magnetics Institute* 2 (8):1-17.

Connor, M. 2004. "The use of triaxial elf magnetic field meter measurements as a predictor of capacity in energy medicine practitioners in a research setting." World QiGong Congress.

Connolly, S., and C. Sakai. 2011. "Brief trauma intervention with Rwandan genocide-survivors using thought field therapy." *Int J Emerg Ment Health* 13 (3):161-72.

Sakai, C. E., S. M. Connolly, and P. Oas. 2010. "Treatment of PTSD in Rwandan child genocide survivors using thought field therapy." *Int J Emerg Ment Health* 12 (1):41-9.

Sebastian, B., and J. Nelms. 2017. "The Effectiveness of Emotional Freedom Techniques in the Treatment of Posttraumatic Stress Disorder: A Meta-Analysis." *Explore (NY)* 13 (1):16-25. doi: 10.1016/j.explore.2016.10.001.

Stapleton, P., A. Bannatyne, H. Chatwin, K. C. Urzi, B. Porter, and T. Sheldon. 2017. "Secondary psychological outcomes in a controlled trial of Emotional Freedom Techniques and cognitive behaviour therapy in the treatment of food cravings." *Complement Ther Clin Pract* 28:136-145. doi: 10.1016/j.ctcp.2017.06.004.

Bach, D., G. Groesbeck, P. Stapleton, R. Sims, K. Blickheuser, and D. Church. 2019. "Clinical EFT (Emotional Freedom Techniques) Improves Multiple Physiological Markers of Health." *J Evid Based Integr Med* 24:2515690X18823691. doi: 10.1177/2515690X18823691.

Jones, J. 2006. "An Extensive Laboratory Study of Pranic Healing Using Contemporary Medical Imaging and Laboratory Methods." Seventh World Pranic Healers' Convention, Mumbai, India.

Jones, J. 2001. "Neurophysiological Measurements of Pranic Healing Using Functional Magnetic Resonance Imaging (fMRI)." Bridging Worlds and Filling Gaps in the Science of Spiritual Healing, Kona, Hawaii.

Chapter 14
The Supramental body

Weiss, Brian L. 1988. *Many lives, many masters : the true story of a prominent psychiatrist, his young patient and the past-life therapy that changed both of their lives*. London: Piatkus, 1994.

Stearn, Jess. 1967. *The Sleeping Prophet the life and work of Edgar Cayce*. [S.l.]: Frederick Muller.

Orloff, Judith. 2010. *Second Sight: An Intuitive Psychiatrist tells her extraordinary story and shows you how to tap your own inner wisdom.* Reissue ed: Random House, USA, Inc.

Frankl, Viktor E. 1992. *Man's search for meaning : an introduction to logotherapy*. 4th ed. Boston: Beacon Press.

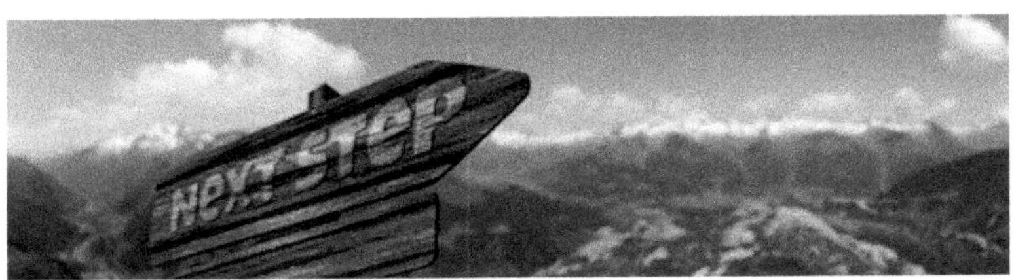

If you have enjoyed reading this book and want more in-depth information about the various techniques described in this book, you might want to have a look at our website for our Newsletter, Blog and upcoming Online Courses and offers. You can also follow **The Quantum Psychiatrist Facebook page** for more information and updates.

http://www.thequantumpsychiatrist.com/
Facebook: @quantumpsychiatrist

Join my free Facebook group at
https://www.facebook.com/groups/quantummentalhealth/

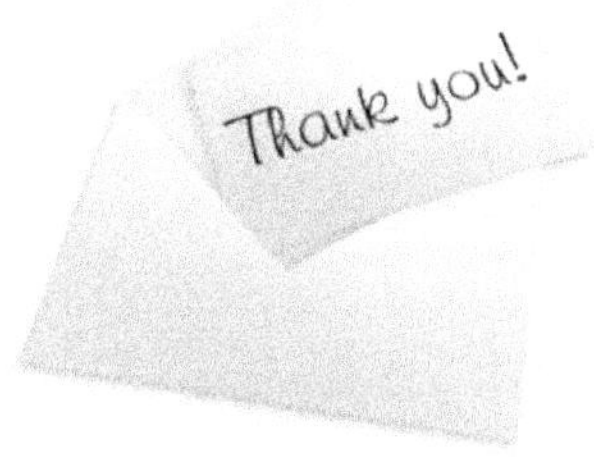

THANK YOU FOR READING MY BOOK!

I really appreciate the time that you have taken out to read this book. I am interested in all of your feedback and I'd love to hear from you!

I need your input to make the next version of this book and my future books better.

Please leave me a helpful review on Amazon letting me know your thoughts on this book.

Thank you!

~ Dona Biswas

ABOUT THE AUTHOR

Dr. Dona Biswas specialised in Psychiatry in India, where she practised for a number of years before moving to Australia. After gaining her Fellowship in Australia, she worked in several reputed public hospitals in Sydney, before moving into her own private practice at Blacktown.

While in private practice, she realised the limited impact that conventional psychiatric treatments were having on her clients' lives and began to train in several cutting-edge interventions to help her clients. She has therefore gained expertise in modalities like neurofeedback, eye movement desensitisation and reprocessing (EMDR), transcranial magnetic stimulation (TMS), transcranial direct current stimulation (tDCS), emotional freedom technique (EFT) and RESET therapy among others and integrates these modalities with conventional treatments in her practice.

She is also an experienced energy healer, being a Reiki Master for more than 15 years and a Seichim Master as well. Her passion is to help people not only overcome their mental illness, but also encourage them to fulfil their untapped and unlimited potential. She works not only with clients with mental illnesses, but also with people who seek to improve their work performance, sense of wellbeing and find meaning in life.

www.ingramcontent.com/pod-product-compliance
Ingram Content Group UK Ltd.
Pitfield, Milton Keynes, MK11 3LW, UK
UKHW020419250726
13967UKWH00007B/2726

9 780648 865100